HOW TO RUN THE
PERFECT
RACE

HOW TO RUN THE
PERFECT
RACE

Better Racing Through Better Pacing

MATT FITZGERALD

PUBLISHING

For my friend Bertrand,
a true pacing master in the marathon of life

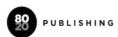 PUBLISHING

80/20 Publishing, LLC
1073 Overland Drive
Midway, UT 84049
www.8020books.com

Distributed in the United States and Canada by Simon & Schuster

Library of Congress Control Number: 2024933842
ISBN 979-8-9892569-4-5 print
ISBN 979-8-9892569-5-2 ebook
Cover and interior design by Vicki Hopewell
Cover photo: Johnny Zhang

CONTENTS

"

It is a misconception to think that during evolution
humans sacrificed physical skill in exchange for intelligence:
wielding one's body is a mental activity."

—TED CHIANG, "UNDERSTAND"

INTRODUCTION

ANOTHER WAY
TO BE GOOD AT RUNNING

My first endurance race was an 8K road run in Dover, New Hampshire, which I completed at age 12 in 1983. My last race (officially) was the 2020 Atlanta Marathon, which I completed while unknowingly infected with COVID-19, the pesky virus that ultimately ended my athletic career. Between these competitive bookends, I contested scores of other road races, track and cross country races, trail ultramarathons, duathlons, and triathlons.

Like any endurance athlete, I had good races and bad races. The good ones included the 2002 Super Run 5K, the 2007 Davis Stampede 10K, the 2009 Palm Springs Half Marathon, and the 2017 Chicago Marathon, where I recorded my fastest times at each of these distances. Then there were the races I won: the 2009 Fiesta Island 10K, the 2016 Lake Chabot Trail 50K, and the 2017 Jailbreak Marathon, among others. But my best race of all was one that I neither won nor ran particularly fast in, and it wasn't even really a race.

While COVID-19 ended my athletic career, it didn't happen right away. For 6 months, I was in the pink, rid of the acute infection and not yet crippled by long COVID, a chronic version of the virus that still afflicts me today. And it was during this last season of health that I ran the race I'm most proud of, albeit unofficially.

The Atlanta Marathon itself was one of my best races. I finished first in my age group and 14th overall with a time of 2:46:59 on a course with more than 1,800 feet of elevation gain. At 48, I was about as fit as I'd ever been, but much of that fitness vanished during the month I spent on my back, coughing up phlegm, bile, and blood. When at last my body gave me the green light to resume exercise, I felt powerfully motivated to reclaim the high perch of supreme conditioning I'd roosted on in Atlanta. While everyone else was complaining about mass event cancellations, I burned to train hard and compete in whatever way I could.

I completed my first tentative post-COVID test run on April 8. The Rambling Runner Virtual Marathon, organized by my friend Matt Chittim, was scheduled to take place 40 days later, on June 17. I signed up. When I tweeted my plan to go from sickbed to start line in less than 6 weeks, a troll replied with the sniping comment, "What could possibly go wrong?" But I had no intention of putting myself through the proverbial meat grinder. Although my goal was undeniably rash, I would play it smart, calling upon my decades of experience to see how fit I could get in such a brief span of time and how well I could perform at an unforgiving race distance despite a severely compressed training buildup.

In concession to both my age and my long history of injury, I designed a program that featured every-other-day running. Each run would count, however, with high-intensity workouts and long endurance runs alternating throughout the build, supplemented by loads of nonimpact crosstraining. I knew going in that there would be days when my body would veto the plan, and when it did, I listened. For example, a 20-miler turned into a 12-miler when it became clear that forcing my way through the remaining distance would have put me in a deep hole. Overall, though, my training went well, culminating in a confidence-boosting 14-mile steady-state run that left me believing a sub-3-hour marathon might be possible.

The nice thing about virtual races is that you get to choose your own route. I chose a 2-mile loop that started right outside my front door, with a makeshift fluid station set up at the foot of my driveway. Never before had I started a marathon with less certainty about what would happen. In previous cycles, I'd built upon a solid base of fitness with 12 to 16 weeks of focused training that rendered me 100 percent prepared to do my best while also supplying me with a very precise sense of what I could do on race day. At the Chicago Marathon, for example, I started out with the goal of running 6:05 per mile straight through, having deduced from key workouts that this pace represented my current limit. How accurate was my assessment? Well, I finished in 2:39:30, which works out to an average pace of 6:05.005 per mile.

Comparatively, the Rambling Runner Virtual Marathon was an exercise in flying blind. Scarcely more than a month earlier, I had struggled to jog 6 miles at 10 minutes per mile, and although I had made rapid progress since then, my goal of breaking 3 hours felt far more like a guess or a hope than a prediction. But that was part of the fun. To achieve the best possible result, I would have to lean on the deep internal knowledge I'd accrued from four dozen prior marathons and *feel* my way to my present limit.

The other nice thing about virtual races is that you get to choose when you start. But with a high temperature of 90°F forecasted in Oakdale, California, I elected to set out at a standard marathon gun time of 7:00 a.m. I was skirting the fenced perimeter of the neighborhood dog park, alive with frolicking canines observed by clustered humans, when my watch chirped. A quick wrist glance revealed a split time of 6:44 for the first mile, 5 seconds ahead of target. To the uninitiated, 5 seconds sounds like a rounding error, but the experienced runner knows that if their target pace represents their true limit, running just a few ticks faster will result in a head-on collision with the wall somewhere down the road.

Yet my pace felt right in a way I can't explain. I somehow *knew* I could keep it up, and there would be no wall, unlike my debut marathon 21 years before, when I'd *thought* I knew I could sustain the faster-than-planned pace I'd started at in a fit of youthful exuberance, only to find myself walking at 19 miles. But I was no longer that runner, and although I couldn't predict exactly how the next 25 miles would unfold, I'd have bet my life savings that I wouldn't walk.

And I didn't. To the contrary, I sped up, completing the marathon in 2:54:52, which equates to 6:39 per mile. I put everything I had into the last 2 miles and eked out my quickest splits, but not by much (6:29, 6:31). The goal of every racer is to finish knowing they couldn't have gone any faster, and I did that in the Rambling Runner Virtual Marathon. It wasn't my fastest race, and I didn't win, but it's the closest thing to a perfect race I've ever run.

THE GREAT EQUALIZER

It is often said that races aren't run on paper. The expression is used to make the point that great preparation does not guarantee a great performance. To fulfill the potential they bring to a race, runners must execute it perfectly, which isn't easy. An honest runner can almost always look back at a completed race and identify errors or lapses that, if avoided, could have saved them a few seconds at least.

Perfection is difficult to attain in all sports, of course. You will never hear the winner of the Wimbledon tennis tournament or the Masters golf tournament claim that they played perfectly. What's different about running, though, is its relative simplicity. In tennis, golf, and other sports, execution has a number of important elements. In running, however, execution is about pacing first and foremost. After all, a race is nothing more than an attempt to get from point A to point B in the least time possible, and the primary determinant of success in this effort is pacing, or how fast you choose to run at each moment throughout the race. There's no better feeling in our sport than running the perfect race, but it is reserved for those who fully master the skill of pacing.

In light of this fact, you would think that pacing skill development would be a major point of emphasis for most runners, but it's not. The typical runner recognizes that pacing matters and knows they need to get better at it yet does little more to improve than vaguely try to do better each time they compete. Mastering the skill requires a more intentional, structured, and sustained approach, as I learned over the course of my journey from youth runner to veteran coach.

HOW I DISCOVERED THE POWER OF PACING

My earliest memory of running longer than the typical playground distance dates back to 1978, when I was 7 years old and living with my family in the deep woods of Hillsboro, New Hampshire. My dad, who at that time ran for fitness (he would later become a marathoner), owned a cool little gadget that he would hook to the waistband of his shorts and use to measure distance when he "jogged" (his word). This pedometer, as it was called, looked like a cross between a compass and a pocket watch and made a satisfying clicking sound with each stride. I had no particular interest in jogging at that age, but I was very interested in Dad's pedometer, so I took it for a spin one day, clicking off a full mile (assuming the thing was accurate).

By the age of 12, under my father's continued influence, I was running regularly, using a cheap children's sports watch to measure time and using various landmarks—mapped out with the aid of the family Renault's odometer—for distance. Numbers weren't the be-all and end-all of the running experience for me, but I liked how they gave purpose to it. A soccer player as well, I saw times and distances as being roughly equivalent to the tally of goals and assists I kept as a striker for the Bobcats of Oyster River Middle School.

In high school, having been forced to quit soccer after I suffered a catastrophic knee injury during a game, I ran cross country and track. Our team's bread-and-butter track workout during the outdoor season was 12 × 400 meters at a roughly 1-mile race pace. My teammates and I made a game of it, each runner taking his turn leading a lap, at the completion of which the others tried to guess the time. We got so good at the game that the winning guess was seldom more than a few tenths off in either direction.

More than a decade later, at 28, I ran my first half-marathon in dragstrip-flat Phoenix. In addition to the usual awards for overall and age-group placement, a prize was given by the race organizer to the runner who came closest to correctly predicting their finish time. I reckoned I was fit enough to average 6:00 per mile, which would yield a finish time of 1:18:39. To take a bit of pressure off myself, I rounded up to 1:19:00, which was unfortunate because my actual time of 1:18:46 would have earned me a gift certificate from a local running specialty shop.

This happened in 1999. By 2001, I was coaching other runners. Like a lot of new coaches, I took my own depth of experience for granted initially. Forgetting I hadn't always known how to pace my running correctly, I was surprised by the kinds of mistakes my clients made. The biggest training error I saw was getting stuck in what I call the moderate-intensity rut—doing way too much training in the no-man's-land between easy and hard. I've since become known for advocating an "80/20" training method, where 80 percent of training is consciously performed at low intensity and the rest at moderate to high intensity.

I also saw plenty of bad race pacing. An example is Chris, whose personal-best marathon time prior to hiring me was 3:13. When his next marathon rolled around, Chris was in 3:05 shape by my estimation, but he ended up running 3:08 after having completed the first 20 miles at a 3:02 pace and then blowing up. As a general matter, I am happy with an athlete's race performance whenever the athlete themselves is happy, but in this case, I must admit I was a little unhappy when, after throwing away roughly 3.2 percent of his fitness,

Chris texted me to say he felt good about losing "only a few minutes" in the last few miles.

"A few minutes!" I wanted to reply (but didn't). "Is that your idea of good pacing?" It wasn't just that Chris had executed poorly. He'd also failed to value pacing properly, shrugging off the loss of "a few minutes" like a billionaire dismissing a few lost dollars. Imagine a boxer being complacent about a few extra punches to the head that could have been prevented with more vigilant defenses or a golfer waving away a few quadruple bogeys that might have been avoided with more careful club selection!

COMPETE AT YOUR FULL POTENTIAL

Pacing is everything in competitive distance running. I mean it: everything. It is the sport's defining characteristic—the singular quiddity that makes distance running different from all other sports and exercise activities, including other forms of running. Take sprinting. The word *sprint* is used rather loosely in colloquial speech, but the true definition of a sprint is a race that is performed at maximal effort from start to finish—which is to say, without pacing. By this standard, there is no such thing as a sprint that lasts longer than 45 seconds, give or take, because it's impossible to minimize completion time in a race lasting longer than about 45 seconds without deliberately holding back a bit at the start. It is pacing that distinguishes a distance event from a sprint. At the other extreme is jogging, or running for exercise, as my dad used to do in his pedometer days. Jogging is also a form of running, but we don't lump it together with the sport of distance running any more than we do sprinting. The difference again is pacing. In this case, whereas the noncompetitive jogger is just trying to fill a certain amount of time with healthy exertion, the competitive distance runner is trying to cover a fixed distance in the least time possible, an objective that demands skillful pacing.

Naturally, some competitive runners are more serious than others, but every runner should take pacing seriously and seek to master the skill. It's a very different sort of commitment than spending thousands of dollars on gear or working out twice a day every day. You don't have to carve out extra time or accept a higher risk of injury to get serious about becoming a pacing master. Like a boxer staying vigilant in their defenses or a golfer taking pains to always select the right club for the next shot, a runner should make every reasonable effort to ensure bad pacing doesn't needlessly limit their improvement. Do you really want to run slower race times than you could just because you can't be bothered to master your sport's most fundamental skill? I didn't think so!

For me, though, pacing's importance goes even deeper. I see it as a democratizing element of our sport. There's nothing you can do about your talent. Whatever genes you were born with, those are the genes you have to work with. But pacing skill is a completely different matter that depends on body awareness, judgment, and toughness—qualities that aren't affected one way or another by innate ability. Sure, the Olympians happen to have all of these things, including raw talent, in abundance, but there are plenty of runners with far less talent who possess just as much of the other three qualities. Indeed, there's no reason the slowest runner in a given race can't be the best pacer. Nor is there any reason you can't find the absolute limit of your potential by mastering the skill of pacing.

Every runner stops getting faster at some point. But pacing is something that any runner can get better at indefinitely. I know I did. Though my VO_2max peaked in my early thirties, my race execution was still rising when I took my final bow as a competitive athlete. No matter how well you executed your last race, there's always a chance you can do even better the next time. So if you're the kind of runner who likes to improve, know that pacing is the one part of running you can improve in for as long as you choose to run.

WHAT WE'RE UP AGAINST

The vast majority of the runners I've coached weren't very good at pacing when I started working with them. And it's not as if poor pacers seek me out. Research shows that most runners pace far from perfectly in races. Why? I'll provide a fuller answer to this question in Chapter 3, but here are the three main reasons:

1. Pacing is hard! Nobody is great at it initially.
2. Experience is the best teacher of pacing skill, and most runners lack the depth of experience that enables masterful pacing.
3. Runners are exceedingly dependent on their devices, and this dependency undercuts the pillars of pacing ability, hindering the development of body awareness, impeding the application of good judgment, and preventing many runners from fully accessing their toughness.

The last of these reasons is the one that really bugs me, in part because it is literally manufactured and hence unnecessary, in part because it's getting worse all the time and in part because I feel somewhat responsible. I've mentioned that I advocate an 80/20 training method as a corrective for the common problem of doing too much training at moderate intensity—which is in essence a pacing error. The method laid out in the books *80/20 Running* and *80/20 Triathlon* and on the 80/20 Endurance web site has helped tens of thousands of athletes all over the world break free of the moderate-intensity rut. Devices such as heart rate monitors and power meters are helpful in this process because they allow athletes to objectively monitor their exercise intensity, making it easier for those who aren't as adept at reading their effort by feel to balance their training intensities appropriately. The problem is that these same athletes risk becoming even more device dependent and less capable of regulating their effort by feel. This wouldn't be a big deal, I suppose, if the devices were as good at making pacing decisions as a human with mastery of this skill, but they aren't, nor will they ever be.

RUN WITH CONFIDENCE

As a coach, I place a heavy emphasis on pacing skill development. In the beginning, admittedly, my method consisted of little more than chastising athletes when they blew their pacing in a workout and patting them on the back when they executed correctly. In other words, the Coach Matt Pacing Skill Development Program, if you can call it that, amounted to little more than exercising the same vague intention to do better next time that many runners get absolutely nowhere with. In my defense, though, I had come of age at a time when pacing wasn't really talked about much because lack of pacing skill wasn't a widespread problem. When the topic did come up with coaches, their stock advice was to relax and let experience take care of it. But with today's device dependency, experience isn't quite the teacher it once was. Recognizing this, I began to put more thought into devising ways to counteract the negative effects of device usage on pacing skill development.

My modus operandi in all of my efforts to elevate my coaching game is to steal from the best. Heck, even the 80/20 method that I've gotten so much mileage out of was stolen from its discoverer, exercise physiologist Stephen Seiler (who very graciously wrote the foreword to *80/20 Triathlon*). Hence my quest to become a better pacing teacher has largely taken the form of an ongoing effort to collect information about the things true pacing masters do that other runners don't and to formulate these observations into techniques and practices that my athletes can implement in workouts and races. I've also delved deeply into the science of pacing, mining it for other tools with potential usefulness in the development of pacing skill. Over time, this grab bag of methods has evolved into a comprehensive approach to mastering pacing.

If I were a more profit-seeking and less honest person, I would tell you that this approach works perfectly in every case—that it transforms even the most inept pacer into an Olympic-grade master in a matter of weeks. The truth is, it doesn't. Like every other skill, pacing ability is not distributed equally across the population. Individual athletes improve by different amounts with the same approach. But what I can say is that *everyone* I work with on pacing does improve, and by a greater amount, I believe, than they would by continuing to muddle along by their bootstraps. And some do in fact achieve full mastery.

What's more, runners of all types enjoy the process. Analytical types who love data enjoy the pursuit of pacing mastery because through it they learn how to use device data more judiciously and also how to use their own perceptions as an additional source of reliable data. Intuitive types who are daunted by technology enjoy the process because it puts them in control of their devices, which become facilitators of, rather than rivals to, their preferred run-by-feel approach. Even those whose progress comes slowly find that the intentional pacing practice I guide them through makes their running more engaging and rewarding. Indeed, from my perspective as a coach, the most satisfying part of the process isn't seeing athletes get better at pacing but watching them start to trust themselves more. Coaching legend Vern Gambetta once tweeted, "The goal in coaching is to develop self-sufficient, adaptable athletes prepared to thrive in the competitive cauldron. Give your athletes the mental and physical skills. Get them to the point where they trust in their preparation and let them go." I couldn't agree more, and in today's environment, I've come to see the teaching of pacing skill as critical to achieving this larger goal.

The key concepts at play here are *self-trust* and *self-sufficiency*. There is no better feeling in the sport of running than that of knowing what you can do and then going out and doing it. That is the feeling I experienced in my post-coronavirus solo marathon, and that is what I want for you. There's always an element of uncertainty in racing, even when you give yourself more than 40 days to go from coughing up bile to attempting a marathon. Some of this uncertainty comes from factors that are beyond our control, like the weather. The rest comes from inside us—doubts about our ability to execute a smart, gutsy performance. When you've mastered the skill of pacing, all of these doubts go away. You still don't know exactly what will happen (what fun would it be if you did?), but you have total confidence that you will not let yourself down. Close your eyes for a moment and imagine what that's like. Now stop imagining and make it happen!

A writer at heart, I couldn't possibly remain content with sharing what I've learned about pacing skill development with only the handful of athletes I coach one-on-one. Inevitably, I got the itch to compose a book on the subject, and here it is. My hope and expectation is that *How to Run the Perfect Race* will do the same thing for you that my hands-on pacing guidance has done for the individual athletes I coach. I'll start out by defining perfect race execution, which is the ultimate goal of pacing. I will then deliver a concise lesson on the science of pacing, which is far more interesting than you might assume but also serves the practical purpose of equipping you with a better understanding of what it means to master the skill. This will be followed by a fuller explanation of the specific obstacles you'll need to overcome to get where you want to go and the most effective ways to overcome them. Next, we'll explore what it looks like to reach the other side of these obstacles—to become a pacing master. The second half of the book gets down to brass tacks, offering specific strategies, exercises, and plans you can use to programmatically improve your pacing in races, workouts, and the training process as a whole.

What this book will not do is solve the pacing problem for you. There is no silver bullet where pacing is concerned. Remember, the desire to have someone or something else do the hard work of pacing for you is what got you into this mess in the first place! You simply cannot become a pacing master without taking responsibility for it. Good coaching can help, and technology has a valid role to play as well, but in the end, it's on you to execute.

There are two ways to look at this responsibility. From one perspective, it's an intimidating burden, but from another, it's an opportunity. The very fact that skillful pacing is hard and that most runners suck at it and wish someone or something else would handle it for them creates an opening for you to become better at it than most of your fellow runners. While others remain resigned to mediocre or poor pacing or vainly hope that they'll get better at it without making any systematic effort to do so, you can leave them behind (literally) by embracing the process I'm about to teach you. I can't make any promises about how far you will get toward perfection as a competitor, but I can promise that you won't regret the journey.

1

Anatomy of a Perfect Race

The men's elite competition at the 2019 Berlin Marathon was not set up as a formal world-record attempt. In prior years, it had been, and with good success. Eight of the previous 10 men's marathon world records had been recorded in Berlin, including the existing record of 2:01:39 set by Eliud Kipchoge the year before. The marquee entrant in 2019 was Kenenisa Bekele, widely considered the greatest distance runner God ever created but who, at 37, was getting a bit long in the tooth and was 3 years past his last major victory. Hired pacers had been asked to take the race out at 2:55 per kilometer (about 4:41 per mile), which would yield a fast but not historically fast marathon time, close to Bekele's personal best (PB) of 2:03:03 if sustained for the full 42.2 kilometers. The prevailing opinion in online fan forums was that Bekele himself would not only fail to sustain it but fail to finish, as he'd done in two of his last four marathons.

On the eve of the event, the soft-spoken Ethiopian told the assembled media, "Overall I have prepared well, although my training period of three months is perhaps rather short for a marathon. This was because of an earlier injury. But I am ready for Sunday and want to show what I can do." Having followed Bekele's career closely from the time he burst onto the international running scene with an astonishing 33-second win at the 2001 IAAF Junior World Cross Country Championships, I read more into these last few words than the casual fan might have done. To me, they signaled that Bekele intended to run very fast indeed and that he wished to show one man in particular "what he could do."

Eliud Kipchoge and Kenenisa Bekele had been rivals since 2003, when the latter nipped the former by 0.35 seconds in a 5000-meter race in Oslo. The pair had met again 19 times thereafter, Bekele coming out ahead in 13 of these races but losing all 4 of the marathons they'd started together. Now in the twilight of his illustrious career, Bekele might have had his last chance to cross a finish line in front of his Kenyan nemesis, but taking down his world record would certainly qualify as the next best thing.

My interpretation of Bekele's pre-race comments was validated the next morning when a small lead pack headed by a pair of striped-vested pacers passed through 5 km in 14:24, well ahead of the stated pace and precisely matching Kipchoge's split from the previous year. In the center of the scrum, a relaxed Bekele looked almost as if he were napping on his feet, waiting for the *real* start of the race. When you've watched a runner compete as many times as I've watched Bekele, you can tell by the subtlest cues if he's got his best stuff on a given day, and I could tell by Bekele's half-lidded eyes that he had good legs on this particular day, and he knew it.

A shrunken lead group passed through 10 km 1 second ahead of Kipchoge's record pace and remained a single tick to the good at the halfway point. I knew this could be no accident. Bekele was going for it! The problem, though, was that Kipchoge had sped up significantly in the second half of his record-breaking performance, and Bekele would have to do the same to snatch the coveted title from his rival. Yet Bekele continued to snooze even after the pacers peeled off, leaving him with only a pair of less heralded compatriots to share the work, and by the time they reached 25 km, the Ethiopian trio had fallen 6 seconds behind the invisible specter of Kipchoge.

Approaching 30 km, and another 4 seconds off Kipchoge's standard, 25-year-old Birhanu Legese launched an attack of his own. Sisay Lemma covered it quickly, but Bekele was gapped. Grimacing, he locked his now wide-open eyes on Legese's back like the threat it was, skipping his next drink bottle to save the fraction of a second that grabbing it would have cost him, but it was no use. The aggressor continued to pull away, shaking off Lemma within a few blocks on his way to passing 35 km with a 13-second advantage on the greatest of all time.

The thing is, Bekele hadn't actually slowed down. In fact, he hit 35 km having recorded his own fastest 5K split of the day, and the grimace was gone.

A nervous glance back from Legese affirmed what, by then, Bekele already understood—the younger man was faltering. Bekele came after him like an assassin. Alone in my home office in California, I began to holler at my computer screen.

Just past 37 km, Bekele overtook Legese with brutal authority, as though the would-be usurper were already forgotten, which in fact he was. Back on world-record pace, Bekele was now chasing someone else, present but unseen.

The next 12 minutes were as thrilling as any athletic spectacle I've witnessed. A famously graceful runner, Bekele ran more beautifully than I could ever hope to describe in those last few solitary minutes on Berlin's Teutonically perfect streets, his trademark sprinter's back kick in full effect, head rocking ever so slightly in small concession to fatigue, checking his watch frequently, as though he heard the television commentators raving about how close it was going to be.

More than beautiful, Bekele's self-sacrificial charge to the finish line was *heroic*, the stuff of legend, an aging champion's all-costs bid to etch one last triumph into his legacy. Bekele shot through Brandenburg Gate at 2:00:39 on the race clock, leaving precisely 1 minute to close the deal. The crowd waiting on the other side went berserk. Wincing with effort, Bekele tried to accelerate but couldn't, for he was already going full gas and had been for some time. The video feed now switched to a camera stationed behind the finish line. I saw Bekele grinding. I saw the clock ticking up, counting down. It was impossible to judge the distance. Could he do it? 2:01:31, 32, 33 . . .

Two seconds. He missed by 2 seconds! That's 0.02 percent. Yet Bekele was far from disappointed by the oh-so-near miss. "I knew I was very close to the record, but I couldn't quite make it," he told reporters at a post-race press conference. "Before the race, I did not expect a world record, so I am very happy to take 80 seconds off my personal best."

As a fan of elite running, I love this performance for its poetry and drama. But as a coach, I see it as the epitome of race execution.

DEFINING THE PERFECT RACE

A perfect race is one that the runner could not have completed any faster. If a runner completes a marathon in 2:01:41, and the fastest time they were capable of achieving on that day is also 2:01:41, then the runner ran a perfect race. That's simple enough. But how do we know if a runner has completed a race in the least time possible?

We don't. Like it or not, we cannot definitively determine whether a runner fulfills 100 percent of their potential in a given race. Of course, there are many cases where it is obvious that a runner has fallen short of their potential. In the preceding chapter, I mentioned that I started my first marathon way too fast and found myself walking at 19 miles. I came into that marathon having recently run a half-marathon in 1:18:46, which according to the Run Fast Coach online calculator predicts a marathon time of 2:44:01. My actual finish time was a far-from-perfect 3:38:40. But when no obvious errors are made in the execution of a race, it becomes a lot harder—impossible, in fact—to determine whether the runner could have squeezed out a few more seconds by doing something differently.

We know enough from the scientific study of endurance pacing, however, to identify race performances that are at least close to perfect. The hallmark characteristic of a "perfect" race is a steady work rate from start to finish. The scientific definition of work rate is energy expenditure over time, measured as calories (or kilojoules) per minute. On a flat racecourse such as Berlin's, work rate closely matches pace. Kenenisa Bekele's 5 km split times at Berlin in 2019 were 14:24, 14:29, 14:37, 14:29, 14:32, 14:26, and 14:20; his momentary speed never strayed more than 1.7 percent above or below the median for the race as a whole. That's about as steady as you can get in a race of such length.

Evidence that a consistent work rate is optimal comes from dozens of studies assessing the relationship between pacing and performance not just in running events but in other types of endurance competitions as well. A 2023 study led by Sabrina Demarie of the University of Rome, for example, found that elite 1500-meter swimmers paced themselves more evenly than less experienced junior swimmers and that steadier pacing was associated with faster finish times at both levels. A prior study appearing in the *International Journal of Sports Physiology and Performance* noted that the closer an individual athlete's first-lap run pace was to their average pace for the four-lap run leg of the 2009 European Triathlon Championship, the faster their overall run time was. That same year, Jo Corbett of the University of Portsmouth reported in the *International Journal of Sports Physiology and Performance* that World Championship track cyclists in the 3 km and 4 km events finished faster overall when there was less variation in speed between their first and final laps.

The data from running events tells the same story. In 2021, a graduate student in exercise science at the University of Maine named Brendan Gilpatrick analyzed results from the previous year's HURT100 ultramarathon in search of correlations between specific pacing patterns and performance. After dividing the finishers into three groups based on how well they placed, he found that the fastest group exhibited the least variation in pace over the course of 100 miles.

The same pattern holds at shorter, more popular race distances. In 2011, Thomas Haney and John Mercer of the University of Nevada, Las Vegas, analyzed data files uploaded to Garmin Connect by 285 participants in two separate marathons. Similar to Gilpatrick, these researchers found that steadier pacing led to faster finish times, with very few exceptions.

Even at the elite level, where the goal is not necessarily to run as fast as possible but to beat as many other runners as possible, less variation in speed is associated with greater success. This was shown in a 2021 study led by Brett Kirby of the Nike Research Lab, who used the personal-best race times of elite male runners entered in the 5000-meter and 10,000-meter events at the 2017 IAAF World Outdoor Championships as a basis for comparing how individual athletes "should" have performed against how they actually performed as a result of their race execution. What he found was that the more time a runner spent above their estimated critical speed (an important physiological threshold above which fatigue builds rapidly) prior to the final lap, the farther back they finished. This finding would not be particularly noteworthy if the runners with the fastest critical speeds had spent the least time above this threshold and finished highest. But in fact, like most championship track events, the two races Kirby analyzed featured significant oscillations in pace at the front, and it was the runners who did the best job of staying within themselves despite these oscillations who performed best, regardless of personal bests.

HERE'S THE FINE PRINT

No runner ever completes a race at a perfectly consistent work rate. Hills, winds, turns, terrain, aid stations, and other runners all but force runners to vary their work rate. Apart from these external factors, internal factors also cause pace to fluctuate. Studies have shown that running at any given speed feels harder on a treadmill than it does outdoors, likely because our bodies don't like to feel locked into a rigidly unvarying speed. This may explain why elite runners never match their speed perfectly to the Wavelight electronic pacers made available to them for world-record attempts. Scientists refer to the gentle undulation in pace that comes naturally to human runners as stochastic variation, which is distinct from the conscious fluctuations that occur during "good patches" and "bad patches"—peaks and valleys in perceived effort that would be foolish to ignore.

For all of these reasons, absolute consistency in work rate is neither possible nor desirable in races. Another caveat to the steadiness principle in pacing is what I call the latitude exception. Simply stated, runners execute seemingly perfect races with more than one pacing strategy. In 2019, Brigid Kosgei used even splits to set a women's marathon world record of 2:14:04 in Chicago, running the first half in 1:07:05 and the second in 1:06:59. Three years later, Eliud Kipchoge used positive splits to lower his own world record, passing the halfway mark in 59:51 in an attempt to break 2 hours (something he'd done previously in a non-record-eligible exhibition) before fading to a second-half split of 1:01:18, which was still good enough to lower his world record by 30 seconds. And in 2023, defending champion Tigst Assefa came to Berlin looking to break Kosgei's women's world record. She started right on pace, reaching the midpoint in 1:06:20, but felt so strong that she sped up from there, using a negative split of 1:05:33 to lop more than 2.5 minutes off the record.

Even when positive and negative splits are used to achieve near-perfect performances, though, variation in pace is highly constrained. Kipchoge slowed down 2.4 percent between the first and second halves of the 2022 Berlin Marathon, while Assefa sped up by 1.9 percent in her record-breaking performance. The average recreational runner, meanwhile, slows by an average of 10 percent in the second half of a marathon.

Another limited exception to the steadiness principle is event specificity. Optimal pacing looks somewhat different at different race distances, a phenomenon that is believed to reflect the disparate causes of fatigue in shorter and longer events. In elite 800-meter races, which take less than 2 minutes for top runners to complete, the winner almost always runs a positive split, cover-

How to Run the Perfect Race

ing the second lap a bit slower than the first. In the longer track events—from 1500 meters to 10,000 meters—a J-shaped pacing pattern is associated with the best performances. Runners start fast, settle in, and finish even faster than they started. Half-marathons and marathons are typically won with even splits or nominally positive or negative splits, and in ultramarathons, everyone slows down, though higher finishers slow less.

Again, however, these exceptions to the steadiness principle are tightly constrained among the top performers. When Athing Mu set an American record of 1:55.04 for 800 meters at the 2003 Prefontaine Classic, her second lap was a half second slower than the first—technically a positive split, but c'mon! And when Jakob Ingebrigtsen set a world record of 4:43.13 for 2000 meters earlier that same year, his split times for the race's five laps did indeed follow a classic J-shape pattern, but just barely (56.67, 56.77, 57.35, 57.33, and 55.00 seconds).

All in all, the one major difference between a poorly or decently paced race and a perfectly paced race is that there is less variation in work rate in the latter.

WHY EVEN PACING WORKS BEST

Having demonstrated to your satisfaction that, minor caveats notwithstanding, consistent pacing produces the best results, I will now address the question that is begged by this reality: Why?

The answer lies in the study by Brett Kirby described in the previous section. As mentioned, Kirby's key finding was that the more time a runner spent above their critical speed prior to the crucial last lap of a championship 5000-meter or 10,000-meter race, the farther back they finished. That's because fatigue happens a lot faster above critical speed, where the body loses metabolic homeostasis, than below it, where homeostasis is maintained. There's only so much time a runner can accumulate above critical speed in a single race before they're toast, and it can't be undone by slowing down.

Suppose your critical speed is 6 meters per second. In theory, a runner could oscillate between 6.2 m/s and 5.8 m/s throughout a race and end up finishing in the same time they would achieve by running steady at 6.0 m/s. In reality, however, this can't happen because the runner will fatigue exponentially faster at 6.2 m/s than they will at 6.0 m/s, hastening exhaustion to a degree they can't make up for by periodically slowing down to 5.8 m/s to regain homeostasis.

The typical trained runner can sustain their critical speed for about 30 minutes. What this means is that races that take substantially less than 30 minutes to complete are performed entirely above critical speed, while races that take substantially longer than 30 minutes to complete are performed entirely below it. Obviously, the effect of crossing the critical speed threshold has no relevance in these shorter and longer races, yet steady pacing remains optimal because it has a lower energy cost than variable pacing at intensities both above and below the critical speed, even when the average speed is the same. This was shown in a study led by Erik Kolsung of the Norwegian University of Science and Technology and published in *Frontiers in Physiology* in 2020. Fifteen elite cyclists completed four rides lasting 20 minutes apiece, two at low intensity and two at high intensity. One ride at each intensity was done at a steady power output, the other at a variable output with a matching average wattage for the full 20 minutes. At both intensities, the total energy cost was higher with variable pacing, as were blood lactate levels, indicating that the cyclists would have exhausted themselves sooner with this pacing pattern had the tests continued beyond 20 minutes.

It's as if each athlete is given a matchbook at the start of a race, and it contains just enough matches to last them until they finish, provided their average burn rate is, say, two matches per minute. When the athlete runs at the highest work rate they can sustain for the full distance, they burn precisely two matches per minute. When they run a little slower, they burn one match per minute. But when they run a little faster, they burn not three but four matches per minute. To avoid draining their supply of matches prematurely, the runner may either stick to the highest sustainable work rate from start to finish or spend 2 minutes running a little slower for every minute they run faster, and you don't have to be John Nash to know which option will result in the faster time.

NOT ALL STEADINESS IS EQUAL

All this talk about steadiness and consistency demands clarification. Stable pacing is not the goal of racing. If it were, then perfect race execution would be the easiest thing in the world. All you'd have to do is start out walking and keep walking at the same steady pace until you finished. What makes perfect execution far from easy is that the true goal of racing is to finish in the least time

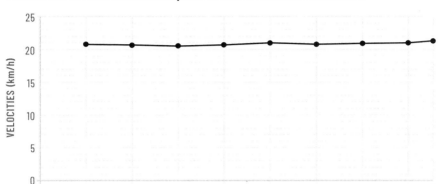

FIGURE 1.1. **Kenenisa Bekele's pace in the 2019 Berlin Marathon**

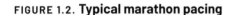

FIGURE 1.2. **Typical marathon pacing**

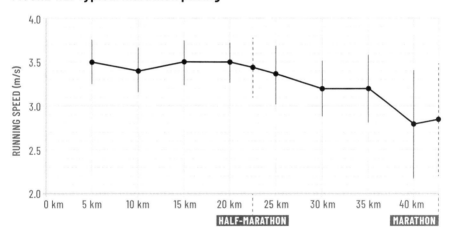

possible, and stable pacing just happens to be a requirement thereof. Of all the paces you might hold steadily in a race, only one will get you to the finish line in minimal time, and that's the pace associated with your highest sustainable work rate for that particular race on that day.

Okay, fine. But how do you know if the steady pace you managed to hold from the beginning of a race to the end was in fact the fastest pace you were capable of sustaining that day? The surest indicator is what I call the *underwhelming finishing kick*. We're all familiar with the phenomenon of the finishing kick (also known as the end spurt). When a runner comes within sight of the finish line, they switch from a paced effort, where they are deliberately running slower than they could to ensure they don't exhaust themselves prematurely, to an all-out sprint, emptying the tank in an effort to shave a few seconds when there is no longer any risk of premature exhaustion.

The speed of a runner's finishing kick depends on two factors. The first is how good they are at sprinting. At all levels of the sport, some runners have a stronger kick than others. The second factor is how tired the runner is when they initiate their kick. The more energy they've saved for the end of the race, the more they'll be able to accelerate. But while a speedy kick is fun to watch, it is actually evidence of imperfect pacing, as Barry Smyth of University College Dublin pointed out in a 2018 study on marathon pacing. After analyzing the split-time data of more than 1.7 million marathon finishers, Smyth found that not only were aggressive starts associated with slower finish times as a result of bonking but fast finishes were "also associated with slower finish times because they sometimes signal cautious pacing earlier in the race, as if runners are holding back for a final sprint." In a perfectly executed race, the runner chooses a steady work rate that leaves them with just enough energy to avoid slowing down on the homestretch or perhaps to pick up their pace ever so slightly, because the few seconds they lose as a consequence of failing to unleash a blistering dash to the line are made up for many times over by the faster pace they maintained from the start.

THE UNSEEN PART OF PERFECT PACING

Figures 1.1 and 1.2 show what a perfectly executed marathon (specifically, Kenenisa Bekele's 2019 Berlin Marathon performance) and a typical marathon look like in graphical form. As you can see, they're very different. However, from the perspective of a marathon spectator standing curbside at the event's 5-mile mark, perfect execution and typical execution look the same. All they see are two runners running.

To fully appreciate what it takes to execute the perfect race, we must peer inside the mind of the pacing master. When we do, we discover three key traits that distinguish runners capable of perfect execution from those not yet so capable: body awareness, toughness, and judgment.

Body awareness (or what scientists call somatic awareness) relates to a runner's feel for their performance limits. Although pacing can be assisted by objective data (as evidenced by Bekele's frequent watch glances), it is done mainly by feel. All competitive runners share a common goal of reaching the finish line in the least time possible. Throughout each race, a single question looms: *Can I sustain this effort level for the remaining distance?* The answer comes not in the form of numbers or words but as perceptions, a continuous evaluation of present levels of effort and fatigue in relation to past experience. That same looming question could also be formulated this way: *Am I feeling how I should be feeling at this point of the race?*

Some runners are better than others at reading these perceptions, and Bekele showed exquisite sensitivity to his limits in Berlin, most obviously when he held steady instead of answering Legese's attack, but not only then. When Bekele said after the race that he did not expect a world record, I took him at his word. Why, then, did he start the marathon smack on record pace? Because every pacing master knows better than to allow expectations to rule their performance. Goals and expectations provide a good starting point for successful race execution, but that's all they do. When the gun goes off and you start moving, you need to be willing and able to adjust your effort appropriately based on external conditions and also on disparities between how you expected to feel and how you actually feel.

For the runner, such adjustments can go in either of two directions. While it's more common to sense the need to dial back one's effort from the expected or desired pace in response to adverse conditions or shaky legs, there are occasional, special races in which the perceptive runner discovers that they are capable of something remarkable, as Bekele did in Berlin. But a single early adjustment is not enough. Optimal pacing is a matter of incessant fine-tuning, as Bekele demonstrated in taking full advantage of the opportunity he discerned when he came out the other side of his rough patch.

Which brings us to judgment. Bekele's decision to let Legese and Lemma get away from him between 30 and 37 km was just that: a decision, and one that not every runner would have made. In his post-race remarks, Bekele revealed that his left hamstring had tightened up when he'd tried to answer Legese's surge, hence the grimace. Although frustrated by the ill-timed anatomical malfunction, Bekele knew better than to resist it, so he shifted his focus from staying with the leader to limiting his losses and remaining in a position to take advantage of

Legese's faltering, should it happen. And it did happen, because Legese had made a mistake—specifically, a pacing mistake—in surging too hard too early in the race. In fact, he wound up finishing more than a minute behind his elder.

To fully capitalize on the opportunity his body awareness and judgment had created, Bekele needed to exercise the third key aptitude for pacing mastery: toughness. Most runners are tough, but Bekele demonstrated a rare kind of toughness in going after Kipchoge's world record in the "I-don't-care-how-much-it-hurts" manner that he did. There is no way to objectively measure how hard one is trying in a race. A runner might feel they tried as hard as they could in a race only to plunge even deeper into the pain cave in the next one, when perhaps there's more at stake. In running, the limit is always mental, the pain tank filling before the gas tank empties,[1] and the tougher a runner is, the closer they can get to their physical limit before they hit their invisible—but no less real—mental limit.

YOUR PERFECT RACE

Kenenisa Bekele is far more talented than you or me. But that's not why he ran a 2:01:41 marathon. He ran a 2:01:41 marathon because he got the most out of his talent by drawing upon his body awareness, toughness, and judgment to execute a perfect race. You and I can forgive ourselves for not being as talented as Bekele, but can we excuse ourselves for not getting the most out of our talent?

There are those who try to excuse setting a low bar for themselves as runners. They look at studies linking steadier pacing with better performance and claim that talent is somehow responsible for both. Google the phrase "negative splits unrealistic for most runners" and you'll see what I mean. The problem with these efforts to justify soft standards for race execution is that science offers irrefutable proof that most nonelite runners pace themselves suboptimally and can do better with a little help.

An ingenious experiment designed by Claire Molinari of the University of Paris-Saclay and published in the *International Journal of Environmental Research and Public Health* in 2021 is one example. Eight recreational runners were asked

---

[1]   There are exceptions—in an all-out sprint, runners do encounter physical limits, and endurance races often conclude with an all-out sprint to the finish line. I'll say more about this phenomenon in the next chapter.

How to Run the Perfect Race

to complete a set of four 3000-meter time trials. The first was self-paced and served to establish a baseline. In the remaining three time trials, the runners were required to maintain a steady state defined by the average speed, the average rate of oxygen consumption, or the average heart rate recorded in the first time trial. Collective finish times were 6.4 percent, 14 percent, and 12.4 percent faster, respectively, in the three steady-state time trials than in the freely paced time trial. The average finish time in the fastest time trial, regulated by oxygen consumption, was 12:20, compared to 14:14 in the freely paced time trial. Same runners, same level of fitness; the only difference was pacing.

The lesson of this study is not that runners should complete each race at a fixed rate of oxygen consumption. That's not how perfect races are executed in the real world (although the physiologically governed time trials did result in pacing patterns that more closely resembled those exhibited by elite runners in middle-distance events). The lesson, rather, is that most runners race a lot slower than they could with science-backed guidance. Honestly, as esoteric as Molinari's guidance might seem, all it really did was force runners to be more consistent than they were on their own and to push harder.

You've come to the right place for science-backed guidance on pacing to help you achieve performance leaps similar to those enjoyed by the runners in Molinari's study. But before we get to that, let's first dive deeper into the fascinating science of pacing and its surprising history.

2

The Science of Pacing

As much as I would like to say I wrote the book on pacing, that honor belongs to Andrew Edwards and Remco Polman, who coauthored *Pacing in Sport and Exercise* in 2011. I did, however, write the foreword to that groundbreaking volume, which I was privileged to read ahead of its public release. More than a decade later, I'm still able to recite from memory the authors' definition of pacing: "The goal-directed distribution and management of effort across the duration of an exercise bout." There's a lot packed into this short statement, including concepts of self-regulation and effort perception that are well worth exploring in depth. But first let's talk about the "goal-directed" part.

Since the beginning, scientific efforts to understand pacing have focused on the concept of the limit, and rightly so. All types of human performance, including running, are defined by their limiters. To understand what stops people from going faster, higher, or farther than they do is to understand how they go as fast, as high, and as far as they do. The thing that makes running, and especially distance running, different from other types of human performance is that the nature of the limiter is not self-evident. In a sprint, the limiter is seemingly obvious: speed. One can dig a little deeper and ask whether sprint performance is limited by how quickly an athlete can turn over their legs or by how much directional force they can apply to the ground with their foot, but such questions are answered relatively easily (turns out, it's the latter). In longer events, the limit is a lot fuzzier. At almost any point in a 1-mile track race or a

100-mile trail ultramarathon, a runner could, if they chose to, run faster than they are. So it's not a speed issue. But if not that, then what? Answering this question is key to unlocking the mystery of pacing. All runners seek their performance limit in races. Pacing is the tool we use to find our limit. But what the heck is the limiter?

IN SEARCH OF THE LIMIT

Science is essentially a formalized effort to overcome bias. It's an effort that never fully succeeds, however, because science is practiced by the same biased humans who seek to overcome their natural biases in practicing it. The quest to understand pacing has been tainted by two biases in particular. The first is an abiding tendency to privilege the physical (i.e., the body) over the nonphysical (the mind). The second is a propensity to overlook the nonmeasurable or not-yet-measurable in favor of the measurable. If not for these twin biases, scientists might have solved the mystery of pacing more than a century earlier than they did.

The first modern theory of human endurance was entirely biological in nature, overlooking the mind altogether. Its creator was Archibald Vivian Hill, who published under the name A. V. Hill and is widely regarded as the father of exercise science. Born in 1886 in Bristol, England, and educated at Cambridge University (where he also ran track), Hill began to study the physiology of muscle contractions in 1909. His interest in the phenomenon was sparked by the then recent discovery that muscles have the ability to contract without a supply of oxygen. Prior to this discovery, oxygen was believed to be an absolute requirement for muscle contraction. Hill's work took the newfound existence of anaerobic (meaning "without oxygen") muscle metabolism as its starting point and yielded many additional discoveries.

In the early 1920s, Hill came up with the concept of oxygen debt, for which he was awarded a Nobel Prize. His key insight was that, although the muscles are able to perform a limited amount of work in the absence of oxygen by turning glycogen (the storage form of glucose in the muscles and liver) into lactate, eventually this lactate has to be turned back into glycogen with the help of oxygen. Hill's own experience on the track (he had a PB of 4:45 in the mile) fed into this realization. He'd always wondered why his breathing rate remained elevated for a few minutes after a hard workout or race and then gradually returned to normal. The concept of oxygen debt helped explain what the body was trying to accomplish through this process.

Hill's next step was to test his insight on athletes, including himself, by tasking them to run around an 85-meter track while breathing into a mask that collected exhaled gases in a bag worn like a backpack. The specific protocol Hill devised required subjects to go faster and faster until they reached exhaustion, a type of endurance test that became known as an open loop because there was no predetermined endpoint. Through such experiments, Hill learned that each person has a maximal rate of oxygen consumption that is highly correlated with their maximal sustained running speed. Today we refer to this limit as aerobic capacity, or VO_2max. All runners consume more oxygen as they run faster, and the fastest runners are able to consume the most oxygen, but even they reach a limit eventually, and exhaustion soon follows.

Hill pegged the heart muscle as the source of this limit. When intense exercise is sustained, he believed, the heart can't supply enough oxygen to the working muscles to meet their energy needs, causing the muscles to make up the balance by turning glycogen into lactate without oxygen. But only so much oxygen debt and lactate can accumulate before the muscles fail, at which point the athlete must slow down or stop so that oxygen can be made available in sufficient quantities to turn the accumulated lactate back into glycogen.

Hill now stood just one small step away from formulating a theory of pacing. He had identified the limiter of endurance exercise—or so he thought. All that was left for him to do was to figure out how athletes manage to reach but not exceed their limit in competition. Oddly, Hill never took this final step. The reason, I suspect, has to do with the open-loop nature of his experiments, where subjects ran at incrementally increasing speeds to the point of failure. This format made sense in that it was the failure point that Hill was most interested in. He wanted to know what caused an athlete to stop when they did. The problem, however, was that there was no self-pacing element in this protocol. The pace was set by the experimenter, not the runner, who was required to keep accelerating on command until they couldn't. This is completely different from an actual race, which is a closed-loop endurance test where each athlete regulates their own pace. Steeped as Hill was in his experimental design, it seems to have never crossed his mind to explain how pacing operated in relation to the hard limit of muscle failure.

Fortunately, the next generation of exercise scientists stepped up to develop a theory of pacing that was consistent with Hill's biological explanation of human endurance. Less fortunately, it wasn't a very good theory. What these midcentury bioreductionists proposed was that athletes somehow automatically race at the highest speed they can sustain without causing their muscles to fail before they reach the finish line. A key contributor to this literally mindless theory of pacing was David Costill, who did his most important work at Ball State University in Muncie, Indiana. In 1978, Costill led an experiment in which lactate levels were measured in 18 runners as they completed time trials and races of various distances ranging from 3.2 kilometers to a marathon. As expected, lactate levels were found to be higher in shorter events run at faster speeds and lower in longer events run at lower speeds. At all distances, however, performance was highly correlated with the subjects' maximal lactate steady-state (MLSS) running speed, or the highest speed each runner was able to sustain in a separate test without going into oxygen debt. On the basis of this finding, Costill's team concluded that "runners may set a race pace which closely approximates the running velocity at which lactate begins to accumulate."

Absent from this study was any effort to explain how runners identify the velocity at which lactate begins to accumulate. One thing is certain: Runners don't wear lactate meters that enable them to stay just below the allowable limit in the same way that motorists use their speedometer to stay below the legal speed limit. This left only two possibilities, assuming Costill's speculation was correct. One was that the brain possessed some sort of hidden internal lactate meter that monitored blood lactate and enforced a limit in the way a thermostat enforces a temperature limit. The other was blind trial and error—an unconstrained process whereby runners find out the hard way how fast they can go without exceeding the lactate limit at each race distance. Neither of these possibilities had any empirical backing. People don't *feel* their blood lactate level the way they feel other things, like body temperature. And as for the second possibility, while it is true that most runners are bad at pacing initially and get better over time, they aren't nearly as bad as we would expect them to be if their pacing decisions were entirely a matter of trial and error.

Another problem with Costill's conclusion that lactate accumulation limits performance at a range of exercise intensities is the fact that, as Costill himself observed, lactate levels vary widely in races of different distances. If lactate really caused muscle failure, it would do so at one specific level. In response to this criticism, believers in a strictly biological model of endurance broadened it to encompass other mechanisms of fatigue. The revised explanation of pacing that came out of this effort proposed that fatigue was caused by different mechanisms in different situations. In a short test lasting only a few minutes, for example, fatigue might be caused by muscle cell depolarization (the same mechanism that causes batteries to fail), whereas in a longer test, it might be caused by a core body temperature increase, muscle damage, or glycogen depletion.

What did not change in this modified model, however, was the general idea that endurance performance was limited by physiological failure. All it did was multiply the types of failure that might occur, and in so doing, it multiplied the pacing problem, offering no answer to the question of how athletes regulate their effort in such a way as to just barely avoid whichever specific type of failure would occur first in a particular event.

But there was an even bigger problem: Endurance performance is not actually limited by physiological failures of any kind. It's true that intense and prolonged exercise causes all sorts of disruptions to biological homeostasis. Lactate levels increase, pH levels decrease, cellular damage occurs, glycogen levels drop, core body temperature climbs, and more. But in study after study after study, researchers found that none of these disruptions ever reached a point where it could have directly forced an athlete to stop exercising involuntarily.

The final experimental nail in the coffin of the biological model of exercise tolerance came in the form of a meticulously designed study by Spanish researchers that appeared in the *Journal of Physiology* in 2015. Its aim was to exercise volunteers to the point of exhaustion in a variety of ways and measure absolutely everything to find out once and for all which specific physiological breakdown, if any, set the limit. Twenty-two subjects performed 10-second, all-out sprints on stationary bikes, recovered fully, and then pedaled at incrementally increasing power levels to failure—not once but on multiple occasions, with new wrinkles added each time. In half of the tests, the subjects breathed regular air, while in the other half, they breathed oxygen-poor air, simulating high altitude. After quitting each test, the subjects rested for either 10 seconds or 1 minute, with either a normal blood supply to the legs or a constricted blood supply, and then repeated the all-out, 10-second sprints. Among the measurements taken during and after each variation were blood lactate level, muscle pH, and adenosine triphosphate (ATP) level (ATP being the muscle cells' fundamental energy currency).

The results showed that neither lack of energy supply to the muscles nor chemical disruptions within the muscles could explain the subjects' quitting. For example, when blood supply to the legs was constricted, the subjects were able to produce more power in a 10-second sprint after 1 minute of recovery than after 10 seconds of recovery, which one would intuitively expect. Yet lactate levels were higher and pH levels were lower after the longer recovery, which was a problem for the idea that either high lactate levels or low pH levels caused exhaustion. Having no other option, the researchers concluded, "At the end of an incremental exercise to exhaustion, a large functional reserve remains in the muscles to generate power, even at levels far above the power output at which task failure occurs."

In lay terms, this means the subjects were physically able to keep exercising at the time they stopped. There was no physiological failure. Crazy, right? But facts are facts. The great thing about science is that, although susceptible to bias, it is self-correcting. Given time, it exposes its biases, opening the door to a truer truth. To the (ironic) credit of science, exercise scientists who believed that exhaustion is caused by physiological breakdown were the ones to prove that exhaustion is not caused by physiological breakdown. Which meant that pacing could not be a physiological process. Which meant that pacing remained unexplained.

COMMON SENSE TO THE RESCUE

A. V. Hill's biological model of exercise tolerance actually fell apart long before the Spanish study just described buried it once and for all. The inability of its proponents to produce a scintilla of proof that endurance performance was limited by any specific physiological breakdown was common knowledge within the field of exercise physiology as early as the 1990s. Then in 1996, a South African medical doctor turned exercise physiologist proposed an alternative model of exercise tolerance, which shifted the performance limiter *from the body to the brain*. Tim Noakes argued that, during exercise, the brain receives continuous feedback from various organs and systems of the body—chemical and electrical information streams that enable the brain to monitor things like core body temperature, blood glucose, and hydration; to assess the athlete's well-being from moment to moment; and to react protectively when necessary. If the feedback coming into the brain signals an impending crisis—hyperthermia, hyponatremia, or whatever—the brain, acting as a kind of governor (hence the model's name: the central governor theory), automatically reduces muscle activation, causing the athlete to slow down involuntarily. And there's your limit—not physiological failure but *the threat* thereof.

Pacing, according to this theory, is all about anticipation. Writing in 2011, Noakes explained, "The goal of pacing is to maintain homeostasis and to prevent a catastrophic physiological failure. Multiple, independent systems in the periphery provide sensory feedback that influences central motor drive from the brain to the exercising muscles. The outcome of this information is the pacing strategy that develops during exercise." The governor, then, is a brain-based mechanism that estimates the maximum speed that can be safely sustained over an expected duration and actively enforces this limit.

The central governor theory made a huge impact, not only within exercise science but also beyond it, influencing endurance coaches and athletes all over the world. It had problems of its own, however. Some critics pointed out that if the central governor existed, then we ought to be able to find it. After all, plenty is known about which specific parts of the brain handle different functions. If you're startled by a sudden movement in the periphery of your vision, blame the amygdala. If you succeed in resisting the temptation to eat a cookie you know you don't need, credit the anterior cingulate cortex. Yet despite rapid advances in functional brain imaging and related technologies, nobody has been able to pinpoint a specific brain structure that holds runners back automatically, by just the right amount, in a race.

Another problem was that the central governor theory completely ignored a little thing called consciousness, assigning no role to the thoughts and perceptions we all experience in our efforts to pace our runs. To the extent that Noakes's theory made sense, it did so for zombies, not humans. In response to this second criticism, Noakes revised the theory to make space for conscious brain operations, but this only opened the door to another criticism: If pacing can't be explained without reference to conscious thoughts and perceptions, what need is there for an unconscious central governor that can't even be found?

Among Noakes's favorite "proofs" of the existence of a central governor that controls pacing was the well-known "end spurt" phenomenon, whereby athletes abruptly speed up at the end of a long race, just when (according to A. V. Hill's model of exercise tolerance) they are presumably nearest to their physical limit. Noakes was certainly right to point out that the strict biological explanation of pacing did not account for this almost universal phenomenon. But in an attention-grabbing 2008 paper published in the *European Journal of Applied Physiology*, a brash young Italian exercise scientist named Samuele Marcora challenged Noakes's own explanation of the end spurt and offered a more human, less zombielike alternative. Marcora's simpler explanation for the end spurt was that athletes use a combination of perceived exertion (a.k.a. perceived effort) and awareness of where they are within a race to make conscious pacing choices that ensure they "save something" for the end, at which point they go ahead and empty the tank. Because runners cannot precisely anticipate how things will stand near the end of a race, Marcora argued, and because finishing the race is paramount, "athletes usually choose a slightly conservative pace for most of the race. Near the end of the race, when the information provided by the conscious sensation of effort at a certain running speed is more reliable, most 'conservative' athletes realize that they can significantly increase running speed without reaching exhaustion before the finishing line, and decide to go for an end-spurt. No additional subconscious intelligent system is needed, just our conscious brain."

In 2009, 1 year after his editorial appeared, Marcora introduced his own theory of endurance limits, which he called the psychobiological model of exercise tolerance. According to this new model, the true limiter of endurance performance is neither the body's functional capacity nor a brain-based protective reflex that keeps us from exceeding our physical capacity but conscious self-regulation, where sensations and behavior are controlled through deliberate decisions made in pursuit of goals.

In a stark break from exercise science tradition, Marcora based his model not on biochemistry but on psychology, specifically on a construct known as motivational intensity theory. Developed by Jack Brehm in the 1980s, motivational intensity theory asserts that people enter into difficult tasks, whether physical or mental, with a certain degree of potential motivation that predetermines the maximal amount of effort they are willing to exert to achieve their goal. If this limit is exceeded before the goal has been achieved, they disengage. Marcora proposed that endurance racing is like any other task in that when an athlete hits the proverbial wall in a race, it is not because the body has encountered a physical limit but rather because the athlete has decided that the effort required to keep pushing is too great. It's not that physical limits don't exist—they're just never actually encountered in the endurance context because one of two things always happens first: The goal is achieved, or the effort required to continue pursuing the goal exceeds the athlete's potential motivation and the athlete backs off by choice.

What makes endurance exercise different from other tasks is the specific form that effort takes. In most everyday tasks, such as desk work and parenting, effort takes the form of a nebulous mix of internal resources such as concentration and willpower. In running, however, the dominant form of effort is *perceived effort*. In a 2010 paper, Samuele Marcora defined this critical concept as follows: "Perception of effort, also known as perceived exertion or sense of effort, refers to the conscious sensation of how hard, heavy, and strenuous a physical task is. This perception depends mainly on feelings of effort in the active limbs, and the sensation of heavy breathing (a type of dyspnea)." I will explain how the brain generates this perception in Chapter 5, but for now, it's sufficient to note that as the intensity of running increases and as fatigue sets in, perceived effort rises, becoming more and more uncomfortable. If running continues, the runner will eventually reach a perceived effort level that they feel is intolerable, at which point they will quit. The true limiter of endurance performance, then, is a feeling.

PSYCHOLOGICAL LIMITS

This is a good place to mention that it's not only scientists who tend to be dismissive of the nonphysical and nonmeasurable. We all are. We are therefore prone to thinking of psychological limits as being less real than physical limits, and yet they aren't. Take pain, for example. Studies of pain tolerance have found that everyone has a limit as to how much pain they can tolerate, even when the pain they are experiencing is causing no physical harm. It's the same with perceived effort, and this is why in open-loop fitness tests, even the toughest runners step off the treadmill before they physically have to.

Psychological limits are admittedly kind of smudgy compared to physical limits. When there's more at stake, pain tolerance goes up. Similarly, when (in psychobiological terms) the potential motivation level is higher, perceived effort tolerance goes up. This has been shown in a variety of studies, including a 2012 experiment by British exercise scientists Alexis Mauger and Nick Sculthorpe in which subjects completed a pair of VO_2max tests, one of which was a standard open loop, where runners kept running faster and faster in incremental steps to failure, and the other of which was a novel closed-loop test, which was fixed at 10 minutes in length. As you will recall from earlier in the chapter, VO_2max is supposed to be a hard physiological limit, and yet the subjects of this experiment were able to achieve 8 percent higher VO_2max scores in the closed-loop test than they did in the open-loop test.

How come? Mauger and Sculthorpe speculated that the subjects were simply more motivated in the closed loop; hence they dug deeper—and I think they're right. Remember, according to Brehm's motivational intensity theory, people tend to disengage from tasks either when they've completed them successfully or when they feel that continuing is not worth the effort. In an open-loop run, there's really no such thing as successful task completion; the only thing you get for continuing to run is greater suffering. But in a 10-minute VO_2max test, you know you're done after 10 minutes no matter what, so it's easy to motivate yourself to give it all you've got.

What's important to note here is that the subjects in this study felt they were working as hard as they could in both tests, even though they were objectively working harder in the closed loop. It is in this sense that maximal perceived effort tolerance represents a real limit that cannot be exceeded in any circumstances, but it's a mutable limit that may align with different physiological measurements in different circumstances, depending on how they affect potential motivation.

In the years since Marcora introduced the psychobiological model of exercise tolerance, he and other scientists have gathered plenty of evidence in support of the idea that endurance races are indeed paced by perceived effort. One example is a study led by Bruno Ferreira Viana of the University of Rio de Janeiro, which was published in the journal *Applied Psychophysiology and Biofeedback* in 2016. Nineteen cyclists completed a stationary time trial that consisted of four laps of 9.9 (simulated) kilometers. Upon completing each lap, the cyclists reported their current rate of perceived exertion (RPE) on a 1–100 scale. Viana's team found that, across all subjects, perceived effort ratings increased linearly and peaked at 100 points at the end of the time trial. This pattern was so consistent that anyone with sufficient math skills who was told nothing about the time trial except what the subjects' perceived effort ratings were after the first two laps would have been able to accurately predict the total distance of the time trial.

Further evidence that perceived effort runs the show in pacing comes from studies involving the use of deceptive performance feedback during time trials. In one such study, experienced cyclists completed four simulated 10-mile time trials, receiving accurate performance feedback on one occasion, no feedback on a second, and inaccurate feedback (either 5 percent better or 5 percent worse than actual) on the other two. Despite these disparate informational environments, the cyclists completed all four time trials in about the same time, indicating that they relied on perceived effort rather than objective information to determine how fast they could really go.

In our age of technological hyperdependency, we are quick to assume that our devices are more reliable than our perceptions. The thing to understand about endurance performance is that perceptions don't just indicate our limits; they are our limits. When you feel you can't run any harder, you can't, and when you feel you can, you can—no matter what the numbers say.

Imagine telling a friend that you feel cold, only to hear your friend say, "No, you're not. It's 80 degrees." You'd probably look at them like they were crazy, and you'd be right to do so, because to feel cold is to be cold, regardless of the actual environmental temperature. It's the same with perception of effort. This perception decides how fast you can go, and no objective metric can be more "right" than this subjective feeling.

REDEFINING THE PERFECT RACE

In Chapter 1, we defined the perfect race as one in which the runner maintains a consistent work rate from beginning to end and is able to speed up only slightly on the homestretch despite their best efforts to wow spectators with a scorching sprint to the line. We are now in a position to add some color to this definition.

FIGURE 2.1. **Rate of perceived exertion in time trials of various distances**

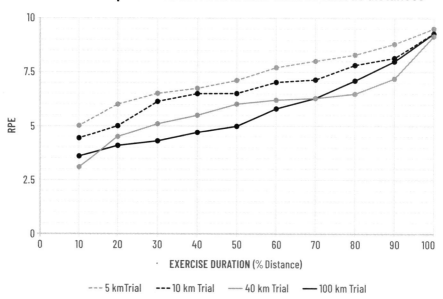

Figure 2.1 is based on a study conducted by South African researchers and published in the *British Journal of Sports Medicine* in 2009. Trained cyclists were given the unenviable task of completing four separate time trials ranging in distance from 5 km to 100 km. At regular intervals, the cyclists were asked to rate their perceived exertion on a scale of 1 to 10. As you can see, the initial RPE was lower for the longer time trials, reflective of the lower work rate that was chosen out of respect for the distance to be completed, but in all four trials, RPE increased linearly and converged at the finish.

Whether or not these time trials were perfectly paced is beside the point. What's certain is that the RPE graph of a time trial or race that was paced perfectly would look a lot like this one. Why? Well, we know that a steady work rate is required to minimize completion time. We also know that RPE increases linearly over time when a steady work rate is sustained. And we know that an athlete cannot exercise beyond their maximal RPE, so they'd darn well better be within sight of the finish when they reach this limit!

In fact, we can be more precise. There's evidence that humans cannot tolerate the discomfort of a maximal perceived effort—the feeling of trying as hard

How to Run the Perfect Race

FIGURE 2.2. **Power output in a 30-second cycling time trial**

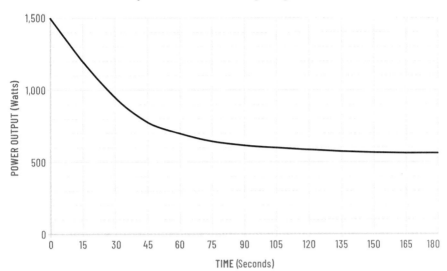

as we possibly can—longer than about 30 seconds. Some of this evidence comes from a cleverly designed study appearing in the *British Journal of Sports Medicine* in 2011. Nine male subjects were asked to complete stationary bike sprints of 5, 10, 15, 30, and 45 seconds. Power data revealed that, despite being instructed to pedal as hard as they could in all five sprints, the subjects held back a little in the 30- and 45-second sprints. The simplest explanation for their noncompliance is that they knew from past experience that they could not tolerate the discomfort of a maximal effort lasting so long, and they therefore paced themselves in the longer sprints without even consciously realizing it.

What these findings suggest is that runners must be within about 30 seconds of the finish line when their perceived effort hits maximum or else they'll need to slow down to keep from exceeding their tolerance. But there's a second reason that runners ought to pace themselves in this way. The graph in figure 2.2 shows the results of a typical 30-second stationary bike sprint. As you can see, even at a true maximal effort, power declines significantly from start to finish. In a 45-second sprint, power would decline further, and in a 60-second sprint, it would fall further still. This precipitous drop has nothing to do with perceived effort but instead reflects physical limits to the sustainability of extreme exercise intensities.

As the sprints keep getting longer, there comes a point where pedaling all-out from the start no longer produces the best performance. In trained athletes, this point comes somewhere between (you guessed it) 30 and 45 seconds. This is why sprinters run all-out from the start of a 200-meter race (which takes around 20 seconds for elite athletes to complete), whereas they hold back a little at the start of a 400-meter race (which takes 45–50 seconds to complete). Putting aside the issue of perceived effort tolerance, a runner who started a 400-meter sprint at maximal effort would—for entirely physiological reasons—slow down so much before the end that they would finish behind an identical clone who paced themselves.

Long-distance races are always paced, of course. But as we've noted, a runner's maximal sprint pace decreases with fatigue. If you want to beat Sha'Carri Richardson in a 100-meter sprint, make her run 20 miles first! Her power will be sufficiently reduced by this prior effort that you just might stand a chance of nipping her at the tape. The fact that maximal work rate decreases over the course of a longer race helps explain why perceived effort increases linearly at any given pace. As fatigue builds, we not only move closer to the limit of how far we can go but also move closer to the (decreasing) limit of how fast we can go, and we feel this.

It's fascinating to see what happens when a runner tries to defy these realities in a race. An example is Sifan Hassan's performance in the 2023 IAAF World Outdoor Championships 10,000 meters. With 250 meters remaining in the last of 25 laps, Hassan burst into the lead. Only Gudaf Tsegay was able to hitch a ride in the Dutch runner's slipstream. As the two women rounded the final bend, Tsegay pulled even with Hassan and raced her shoulder to shoulder down the final straightaway. So closely were the rivals pressed together that Hassan accidentally elbowed Tsegay in the chest, not once but twice.

But that's not why Hassan fell. Track and field fans who don't understand the science of human endurance limits studied the replay over and over, looking for a toe stub or contact between Hassan's and Tsegay's feet, but there was none. Fifty meters from the finish, Hassan simply pitched forward and hit the deck.

The popular term for the phenomenon that caused Hassan to lose the race is "tying up." Studies involving measurements of entropy (or disorder) in the running stride shed light on what happens when a runner ties up. When applied to motor skills like running, entropy indicates how much variation, or "play," there is in an athlete's movements. Researchers have learned that entropy tends to be higher in well-trained runners and when runners are not fatigued, indicating in both instances that they are far from their limit and able to move freely. But when an athlete nears the point of exhaustion, entropy suddenly drops, and their movements become rigid and robotic. The term "tying up" came into use long before it was technically feasible to measure stride entropy, but it perfectly captures what is happening.

In most cases, entropy drop is not visible to the naked eye, but in the most extreme cases, it is. Interestingly, these cases almost always occur in world-class runners who attempt to sustain a protracted sprint at the end of a 5000- or 10,000-meter track race with a medal on the line. We saw it happen to Sifan Hassan in the 2023 World Athletics Championships 10,000 meters, and it happened previously to Steve Prefontaine in the 1972 Olympic 5000 meters, where the replay shows the American suddenly jolting and hinging forward on the final straight as though shot from behind by an unseen sniper, coming almost to a dead stop some 10 meters from the line and losing his bronze-medal position to Ian Stewart of Great Britain.

It's not known exactly what's happening physiologically when a runner ties up this badly. We know that entropy drop causes the tie-up, but what causes the entropy drop? It's a difficult question to answer, for it is virtually impossible to exercise a runner to the point of true physiological failure—the kind we saw in Hassan at Budapest—in a laboratory environment. As I've suggested, the phenomenon occurs only when extremely fit, supremely motivated, and extraordinarily tough runners try to sprint for longer than 30 seconds on tired legs, which tells me that these conditions are absolute requirements for a catastrophic tie-up. But judging by appearances, I suspect it is triggered by some kind of self-protective interruption in the transmission of motor signals from the brain to the muscles, not unlike a power surge tripping a circuit breaker.[1]

---

1   The elusive central governor? Not quite. Brain-centered mechanisms are known to cause involuntary muscle failure in certain special circumstances. The best examples are hyperthermia and exercise-induced muscle cramping. Tying up, I propose, is one more. This is different from Noakes's theory, which proposes that brain-centered mechanisms enforce performance limits in all circumstances.

Few runners appreciate the importance of timing in stride mechanics. Runners would fall all the time if not for an exquisitely synchronized choreography of muscle contractions and relaxations that keep them upright and moving forward. One small interruption throws a spanner in the works that brings the whole system crashing down.

Have you ever seen a professional juggler screw up? If you have, then you know they never drop just one plate but always all 10. Tying up is like that. When the timing is lost, everything is lost.

It's likely that Sifan Hassan would have lost her duel with Gudaf Tsegay even if she hadn't fallen. But she'd still have taken silver. Instead she peeled herself off the track and trotted dazedly across the line in 11th place. It's brutal to say so yet true nonetheless that Hassan ran a less-than-perfect race in Paris. It takes a very special athlete, however, to commit the particular pacing error she did—special enough that, more often than not, they'll get it right, as Hassan did just 6 weeks later at the Chicago Marathon, where she came from behind to win with the second-fastest women's marathon time ever (2:13:44). Nevertheless, her collapse in Budapest puts the final touch on our definition of a perfect race. Simply put, had Hassan fallen 50 meters later, she'd have run the perfect race.

Another brutally honest true statement is that, unlike Hassan, the vast majority of runners truly suck at pacing. Let's find out why and what can be done about it.

3

Why You Suck at Pacing

In 2016, Scottish anthropologist Michael Crawley relocated to Ethiopia for 15 months to study the country's elite running culture. A talented runner himself, Crawley did most of his fieldwork literally on the run, trying and very often failing to keep up with his subjects. But even when he couldn't keep up, things had a way of working out.

One day Crawley was running alone on a gravel road east of Addis Ababa, having once again lost contact with his training partners, when he was caught from behind by a stranger in Adidas racing flats who, instead of overtaking Crawley, offered to run with him. The Scotsman demurred, citing the need to take it easy, but the stranger was having none of it and pressed Crawley to name his preferred pace, promising that whatever it was, he would make it happen.

"Four minutes per kilometer," Crawley conceded.

"Perfect," said the stranger, who was not wearing a watch.

"No GPS?" Crawley asked, dubious.

"It is in here," the stranger said, pointing to his temple.

Sure enough, the next kilometer was completed in 4 minutes flat. It was then that Crawley learned his companion was formerly a professional race "rabbit" who had twice paced his countryman Haile Gebrselassie to marathon world records in Berlin.

If every runner were capable of banging out a precise 4-minute kilometer on command, Crawley wouldn't have considered this story worth telling. In fact, though, few runners possess the pacing chops to replicate the show put on by Gebrselassie's former wingman, which Crawley duly recounted in *Out of Thin Air: Running Wisdom and Magic from Above the Clouds in Ethiopia*. After reading the book, I experienced a kind of counterpoint to Crawley's encounter that served as further evidence that pacing masters are the exception, not the rule. It happened during a virtual running camp hosted by my friend Greg McMillan. On day 2 of the 3-day affair, the campers completed a challenge that required them to run a mile at their individual lactate threshold pace without consulting their watch. Afterward we gathered online to share the results, and they weren't pretty. One runner was off the mark by 40 seconds, while another confessed to peeking at her watch halfway through the challenge, powerless to resist the force of habit. Even the winner was off by several seconds.

All fun and games, though, right? Wrong. The pacing feat that Michael Crawley witnessed on a gravel road east of Addis Ababa wasn't just some frivolous party trick. Nor was the inability of Greg McMillan's campers to judge their pace accurately a matter of inconsequence for their training and racing. To the contrary, a runner who is able to run an exact 4-minute kilometer upon request is a runner who is also capable of executing better workouts and realizing their full potential in races.

Good pacing is all about accuracy. To find your absolute limit in a race without exceeding it is to score a bull's-eye of sorts. It is only to be expected that the runners who succeed most fully in this effort are also, like Michael Crawley's pacing angel, really darn good at measuring things by feel when they run. But pacing skill is difficult to appreciate. When a professional soccer player boots a free kick over the heads of opponents arrayed in a defensive wall, past the outstretched hands of a diving goalkeeper, and into the upper right corner of the net from 30 yards away, we say, "Wow," amazed by the precision with which the player is able to control their body in space. A perfectly executed race is rather dull by comparison, yet pacing is no less a matter of controlling the body in space than kicking a soccer ball, and precision in this skill is no less impressive to those who understand its underlying similarity to other sports skills. Feats like Crawley's companion's 4-minute kilometer hint at how good the best pacers really are—not only when showing off for visiting ethnographers but also in real competition.

I'm not suggesting you have to achieve uncanny exactitude in measuring your runs by feel to find your limit in races. I'm just trying to establish how far away most of us are from pacing mastery. For every retired race rabbit dropping 4-minute kilometers on command, there are two dozen McMillan Running Camp participants missing their 1-mile time target by 40 seconds, give or take. To put it bluntly, the majority of runners suck at pacing. Odds are, *you* suck at pacing. (Or did you pick up this book accidentally?) As to why pacing mastery is so rare, I see three main reasons, none of them insurmountable.

REASON #1: PACING IS HARD!

Snowboarders who lack the ability to execute a triple cork don't beat themselves up for it. Why not? Because it's one of the most difficult snowboard tricks ever invented, and only a handful of boarders on earth can pull it off. Watch a few clips of triple corks on YouTube, and you will see how hard it looks. Pacing, on the other hand, doesn't look hard at all.

As they say, however, looks can be deceiving. A marathon, for example, is a race of roughly 55,000 steps. Completing a marathon in the least time possible requires that a runner execute every single one of those steps at a speed that contributes to this goal. The precision involved in optimal marathon pacing is about equal to that of the 2021 landing of NASA's automobile-sized *Perseverance* spacecraft on a 20-square-mile target located inside a crater on the planet Mars, some 250 million miles from Earth. Except NASA's engineers had mathematics and physics to go by, whereas runners must literally feel their way to this level of preciseness.

Neuroscientist Vincent Walsh of the Institute of Cognitive Neuroscience has argued that piloting the body through an endurance race is among the most difficult tasks the brain can perform, subjecting our most vital organ to the simultaneous demands of driving maximal levels of motor output, managing crisis-level discomfort, and handling the immense cognitive and perceptual challenge that pacing presents. We tend to think of sophisticated mental operations such as landing a spacecraft on Mars as requiring more brainpower than athletic challenges like running 50K trail running events. But in fact the opposite is true, because an endurance race entails both mental work and physical work, and physical work is mental work. As science fiction writer Ted Chiang wrote in the novella "Understand," "It is a misconception to think that during evolution humans sacrificed physical skill in exchange for intelligence: wielding one's body is a mental activity."

It is a proven fact that cognitively demanding tasks, such as taking a math test, result in high levels of brain fatigue. Know what else is cognitively demanding? Pacing a running race.

Science has also demonstrated that sustained efforts of emotional regulation—things like trying to stay calm in stressful situations—produce high levels of brain fatigue. If you have ever done a running race, you can attest that chasing your limit is also a sustained effort to regulate emotion.

Research has shown as well that exhaustive physical work produces high levels of brain fatigue. Would you agree that "exhaustive physical exercise" is a good description of a running race? Thought so.

Finding your limit in a running race is like taking a math test, trying to keep calm in a stressful situation, and working to exhaustion all at the same time, taxing the soggy, electrified, 3-pound organ that makes us who we are more severely than just about anything we experience in our everyday lives. That's hard!

REASON #2: EXPERIENCE MATTERS

Around the same time Michael Crawley was being paced through a long run in Ethiopia by a former professional race rabbit, I was trying less successfully to pace my nephew Caleb through the High Street Hustle 1K Kids Run in Salem, Oregon. My brother Josh had asked me to run with his 6-year-old while he accompanied Caleb's younger brother, Luca. Minutes before the start, I gave my young charge a brief strategy talk.

"Don't go out too fast," I cautioned. "All the other kids are going to take off at full speed and blow up. If you start a little slower, you'll pass them up at the end. Got it?"

The hint of impatience I picked up from Caleb's shrugging promise to heed my advice struck me as slightly ominous. Sure enough, when the horn blared, my nephew took off at a dead sprint, right along with everyone else. The fastest kid in his soccer league, Caleb shot ahead at a velocity that demanded a real effort on my part to match. Recognizing that, at this point, experience would probably be his best teacher, I kept a half step behind him as he pursued the leader, an 8-year-old dressed in a super cool lime-green racing kit with jagged black stripes.

Caleb's chickens came home to roost at the traffic cone marking the halfway point. His breathing became audible, his pace slowed, and he looked up at me two or three times with an uncertain expression. *This could get ugly*, I thought. And it did. Caleb's wheezing intensified to the point I feared he might have an asthma attack (even though he doesn't have asthma). He put up a brave fight, I must say, mustering two or three kamikaze surges before crossing the line second in a very respectable time of 4:42.

If you're smiling right now, it's because you've seen children, either yours or someone else's, endure the same ordeal—or because Caleb reminds you of yourself in your first race. Poor pacing, particularly the pacing error of starting too fast, is the signature first-time endurance racer's error, an almost universal rite of passage.

No human is born a pacing master. Sure, some runners have a greater knack for pacing than others do, but even the most naturally skilled pacers require plenty of practice to achieve true mastery. Through repetition, runners get better at comprehending abstract distances, develop a subtler sense of time, become more skilled at reading their perceptions, learn more effective ways of tuning their attentional focus, and gain a better feel for their physical and mental limits—all of which contribute to more effective pacing.

Research suggests that the last of these elements comes first—that new runners often develop a better feel for their limits before they get better at the cognitive elements of pacing. This was shown in a study performed by Australian researchers and published in *Pediatric Exercise Science* in 2013. Thirteen children between the ages of 9 and 11 were asked to run an 800-meter time trial on three separate occasions. Because this was a novel task for the children, it was expected that their performance would improve across the three time trials through refinements in their pacing execution.

And improve they did—but not through better pacing. Rather, in all three time trials, the children started too fast, slowed down significantly, and then sped up again toward the end. The true reason for their improved performance was simply that *they tried harder*. The 800-meter race distance is notoriously painful. Having never before experienced this particular flavor of suffering, the children were undoubtedly alarmed by the sensations they felt in the first time trial and thus regulated their pace in a way that kept their discomfort from becoming intolerable. But there was nothing solid or impenetrable about this self-imposed limit. In the second time trial, therefore, understanding at least tacitly that they could run a little faster if they were willing to suffer a little more by trying a little harder, they did. The new limit thus established was no less a matter of choice than the first, however, so in the final time trial, the kids ran faster still at the cost of even greater discomfort.

Other studies indicate that athletes continue to home in on their true limit through subsequent stages of athletic development. In Chapter 2, I described research showing that experienced runners exhibit a higher degree of entropy, or "play," in their stride than novice runners but that entropy decreases in all runners, experienced and novice alike, when they near exhaustion. This measurable "tying up" of the running stride indicates that a runner's movements have become highly constrained by proximity to one or more physiological limits. What's most interesting about this research is that, although experienced runners start off with more stride entropy, they typically achieve lower entropy levels and persist longer at minimum entropy in exhaustive running tests, evidence that these runners are able to get closer than less experienced runners to their physiological limits. All runners feel they're at their limit when they quit such tests, but the entropy research tells us this feeling has greater correspondence to objective reality in expert runners.

Mastering the skill of pacing requires not only that you have a good feel for your limits but also that you can measure a mile or a minute accurately without a GPS or a chronometer. In other words, it requires that your perceptions of time and distance be well calibrated to reality, for the goal in racing is to find your limit not in any abstract way but within specific time and distance parameters (e.g., running 13.1 miles faster than ever before). Evidence that experienced runners benefit from well-calibrated internal chronometers can be found in a study conducted by Spanish and Chilean researchers and published in *Motor Control* in 2020. Thirty-eight endurance runners and 39 soccer players were asked to estimate elapsed time (i.e., how long they'd been going) during a bout of sustained running. Among the runners, who of course were accustomed to sustained running, the average error margin was 33 seconds, whereas the soccer players, who, although plenty accustomed to running, were not accustomed to sustained running, missed the mark by more than 2 minutes on average, validating the authors' hypothesis that "temporal and spatial perception can be considered as a cognitive skill of endurance runners."

An even subtler aspect of pacing skill has to do with what runners (and other endurance athletes) pay attention to when racing. Pacing masters know when to tune in and when to tune out during competition—others not so much. Proof comes from a study led by Manhal Boya of the University of Essex and published in *Medicine & Science in Sports & Exercise* in 2017. In this experiment, eye movements were tracked in a mixed group of novice and experienced cyclists while they completed a 10-mile time trial with access to visual feedback on speed, distance, power output, heart rate, cadence, and time. The results revealed a strong association between performance in the time trial and where the cyclists' eyes went while doing it. The faster-finishing experienced cyclists focused mainly on their speed ("How am I performing?") and paid little attention to any other metric besides distance, while the novices scattered their attention more broadly, with distance ("How long until I can stop?") getting the bulk of their eye time. The conclusion that Boya's team drew from these findings was straightforward: "Experienced cyclists are more selective and consistent in attention to feedback during [time trial] cycling."

Relax. You don't need to *figure out* how to be more "selective and consistent" in your "attention to feedback" during running. The whole idea is that all of these things—becoming more selective and consistent in attending to feedback; getting better at measuring time, distance, and speed with your brain; and improving your ability to perceive how hard you're working in relation to your limit—happen naturally as the miles pile up. You don't have to *make* these changes happen; you just need to *let* them happen by continuing to run. This is not to suggest you can't accelerate pacing skill development through various active measures; you can, and I will describe some of these measures in later chapters. It is only to say that, for the most part, the process is unconscious, requiring no less and no more than that you keep running.

Consider the marathon, a famously difficult pacing challenge. The vast majority of participants in any given marathon hit the wall, slowing down dramatically in the last few miles. But not all categories of runners are equally prone to bonking in marathons. In 2017, Swiss exercise physiologist Beat Knechtle teamed up with Pantelis Nikolaidis of the Exercise Physiology Laboratory in Attica, Greece, to analyze pace data from more than 300,000 participants in the New York City Marathon between 2006 and 2016. Among their key findings was that older runners paced themselves more evenly and slowed down less than younger runners with equal finish times, an indication that they had learned through experience how to avoid a late-race fade.

If you've ever doubted your ability to become a pacing master, take heart from the example of Laura, a masters runner I met through Facebook. Laura's first six marathons ended in major bonking episodes. When she signed up for marathon number seven—the 2018 Rehoboth Seashore Marathon—she was resolved to break the pattern. More than just resolved, though, Laura was ready. Her failure to maintain a steady pace in those first six marathons had given her the experience she needed to know how fast was too fast for her in a race of this distance and also how she should feel at different points of a marathon if she was to avoid having to slow down near the end. "I was determined to break 5 hours," she told me afterward via Facebook. "I took it on very deliberately. I wore a pace bracelet for a 4:55 finish. I stuck to the pace for the first 13 miles. My plan was to check in at miles 13, 16, 20, and 23. If I felt good, I would pick it up a notch. At each juncture, I felt great. By mile 16, I was passing people at regular intervals. At 23, I still felt good. I decided there was no way I would allow myself to finish feeling good, so I started to run hard enough to feel the pain." Having reached the halfway mark in 2:22:56, Laura negative-split the second half and crossed the finish line in 4:42:47, a newly minted pacing master.

One thing about experiential learning is that it is aided by an early start, which in running is becoming less and less the norm. Among the several reasons runners aren't as good at pacing today as they were when my dad was doing marathons is that they're taking up the sport later in life. The typical marathoner during the first running boom was someone who ran competitively in high school and kept going, but nowadays runners like Laura—who ran on and off in her late twenties and thirties but only got serious in her forties—are far more typical. Still, examples like hers prove that any runner is capable of using experience to pace themselves ever more skillfully.

REASON #3: DEVICE DEPENDENCY

In July 2020, fitness device manufacturer Garmin fell victim to a ransomware attack that completely shut down the company's online services for several days. Runners and other athletes who relied on these services for uploading and downloading workout data had to make do without them during this period. A disconcertingly large number of the affected athletes responded to the disruption by completely freaking out, many publicly. A Garmin user myself, I did not freak out, but I did appreciate the panic I observed on social media as a reminder of how dependent runners have become on their fitness devices.

Not that I needed reminding. As a coach, I see daily evidence of the stymieing effect sports watches are having on pacing skill development. Here are a few examples of device overdependence I've collected from athletes I've worked with. Not all of them are specific to pacing, but each is representative of a general relationship between athlete and device that holds the athlete back from achieving pacing mastery.

Example 1: Anything for the Score

Icy roads forced Sergio to go slower than normal in the run he'd downloaded to his device from an 80/20 training plan. As he neared the end of the run, Sergio glanced at his watch and discovered that, because of the slow pace, he was not going to achieve the predicted Training Stress Score (TSS, a proprietary metric that factors together workout intensity and duration). To avoid this perceived failure, Sergio extended the run by several minutes, stopping only when the forecasted TSS had been reached, believing that in so doing, he had salvaged the original intention of the run. The problem with this logic was that it assumed Sergio's slower-than-normal pace indicated a lower-than-normal intensity when in fact the extra muscle work needed to remain upright made the effort harder, as he could plainly feel. By extending the run, Sergio made it harder still—all because he trusted an esoteric mathematical projection more than he trusted his own perceptions or common sense.

Example 2: Slave to the Segment

Ryan, a mountain runner I coached for a couple of years, ran the first part of a long, uphill tempo effort much faster than he was supposed to, and he soon paid the price, practically crawling to the summit. When I asked him during our next weekly call what the hell had gotten into him, Ryan admitted that the first part of the climb was a Strava segment he wanted to capture. "Forgive me," I said, my voice dripping with sarcasm, "I didn't realize Strava was coaching you now."

Example 3: Data or It Didn't Happen

While vacationing in the Napa Valley with my wife one summer, I received an unexpected call from Bob, a triathlete I coached. The few such calls I'd gotten from Bob previously had brought bad news, so I was braced for another injury report when I answered. I needn't have worried. Evidently, Bob's power meter had died at the beginning of a bike ride, and he was now standing at the side of the road, wondering if he should go ahead and complete the workout sans data or push it back a day and try to get the device fixed in the meantime. Hearing this, I couldn't decide whether to laugh or cry. In what possible universe could a dead power meter be considered a reason to miss a workout?

Example 4: Virtual Reality Takes Over

Amir completed a set of speed intervals on his indoor bike. Minutes later, my phone notified me that the workout had been uploaded. When I analyzed the data, I saw a massive spike in power at the start of each interval before Amir settled back into the correct wattage zone. Knowing the answer, I asked Amir what was behind those crazy spikes. Can you guess? Bingo! Noticing a lag between the time he started each interval and the time his bike's power meter caught up with the change in output, Amir had pedaled like mad in the first few seconds in a desperate effort to produce the desired number, then slowed down on discovering he'd overshot the target—not once but 12 times in a row. Amir's a smart guy. On some level, he knew his power meter was lying to him, giving him yesterday's news, so to speak. Yet he acted as though he believed the number on the computer was more real than what his body was doing.

Example 5: My Heart Rate Monitor Says I'm Dying!

Kevin posted a concern about his recent training on an online forum that I moderate. Lately, he explained, his heart rate had been a little higher than normal in relation to his pace, and the VO_2max estimates his watch fed him after each run had dipped slightly. A newer runner, Kevin was becoming discouraged and beginning to doubt the effectiveness of the 80/20 method he was following. Having seen this movie before, I asked him how he actually felt while running and whether he would notice anything different if he ran without his watch. "Now that you ask," he replied, "I think I feel fine while running, maybe even good, but when my pace is right and my heart rate seems high, I feel down about it and frustrated during my run and also after." It was just as I had suspected: Kevin's supposed crisis of fitness was in fact a matter of perception, an emotional panic triggered by information that had various possible explanations, all of them more plausible than the one Kevin had assumed in defiance of how he was actually feeling and performing.

Example 6: Happy After the Fact

Suzanne was crestfallen at the end of her tempo run, having fallen short of the pace targets I'd given her. But later, when she reviewed her power data, Suzanne saw that, according to this other metric, she'd actually performed better than her device's estimation of her current fitness level. Windy conditions, I concluded, were the cause of the discrepancy between Suzanne's pace and power numbers. In any case, she was no longer disappointed. Mind you, nothing had changed about the run itself.

I could give you many more examples, but I trust I've made my point, which is that device overdependence is extremely pervasive among runners and manifests in myriad ways. Despite superficial differences, these several examples have one thing in common, which is a certain tension between what the runner's body and mind are saying and what the runner's device is saying. In matters of pacing, this tension takes the form of a disagreement between what feels right to the runner and the runner's interpretation of device data. Each such disagreement must be resolved one way or the other. It's a matter of who gets the final say, the runner or the device. Runners who are comfortable overruling their devices are not overdependent and have a clear runway toward pacing mastery. Runners who are not comfortable overruling their device are overdependent and must gain the upper hand in their relationship with their device to become a pacing master.

Running devices aren't bad. They just aren't as capable of guiding runners to their limit as runners themselves are. That's because (as I mentioned in the preceding chapter) a runner's performance limit is not determined by anything

FIGURE 3.1. **Device overdependence**

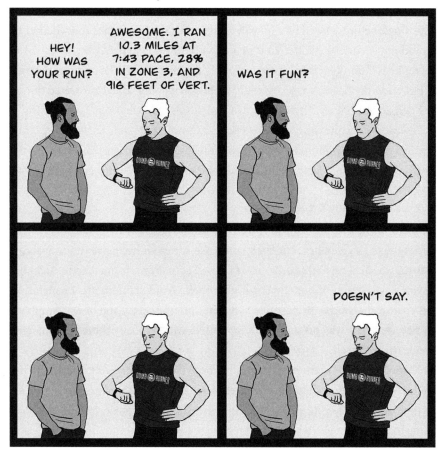

a wearable device can measure. It is determined by subjective perceptions. If a runner lacks sufficient confidence in their feel for pacing and can't grant it the deciding vote in all pacing decisions, pacing mastery will elude the runner, at least for now.

It doesn't stop there, however. Running devices also rob runners of existing pacing ability through a phenomenon called cognitive offloading. Technologies such as running devices become extensions of the brain. We use them to off-load cognitive tasks from our brains to external gadgets. The problem is that when the brain stops performing a certain task that has been assumed by a gadget, the brain gets lazy and loses the ability to perform the task for itself.

For example, research has shown that habitual reliance on GPS technology for navigation causes spatial memory to deteriorate and leads to measurable atrophy in the hippocampus, a part of the brain that's heavily involved in helping us find our way around. Running devices do something similar with respect to pacing skill. The more we lean on them in our pacing decisions, the worse we get at reading our perception of effort; measuring time, distance, and velocity by feel; and knowing our limit.

Too big to ignore, the problem of device overdependence has gotten the attention of scientists. In 2020, the journal *Psychology* published a study led by Pierluigi Diotaiuti of the University of Cassino and Southern Lazio in Italy. A group of 111 runners supplied information about their use of "sports trackers" and completed a questionnaire designed to assess device dependency, which was scored on the basis of how subjects answered questions such as, "If you could not have your device with you, would you still train?" The results indicated that most runners start off relying too much on their devices. While some worked their way past their overdependence, others didn't.

In particular, runners who managed to escape device dependency tended to pass through clear stages in their use of sports trackers. The first stage was one of exploration and discovery—learning what their device could do, essentially. From there, runners moved into a consolidation phase, characterized by a more focused and purposeful use of key features. Then came the paring phase, marked by a rigorous selection of features that left runners attending only to data they deemed essential to goal achievement. The authors concluded that "more experienced runners . . . have shown that over time they have acquired a progressive mastery and internal control of their performance functions," and they were able to use "the sport trackers in a strictly instrumental way, for which there was no perception of dependence or submission."

Like I said, it's all about who has the final say, the runner or the watch. Runners who aren't comfortable overruling their device lack agency in their training, whereas those who get to the point where they trust themselves more than their watch gain a firm hand on the tiller of their running experience. Although this study did not look at specific consequences of device overdependence, I would bet my life savings that, as a group, the runners in this study who were least dependent were the best pacers.

A second noteworthy study on training device usage by runners was performed by scientists at the University of Twente and published in the journal *Sensors* in 2021. Through a combination of interviews and diaries, 22 competitive recreational runners provided detailed information about how and why they used their training devices. A number of these runners had interesting things to say about the tension they experienced between their own opinions and those of their device concerning pacing matters. Their natural inclination was to turn over control to their device and run on autopilot, as it were. But what they discovered was that their gadgets weren't all that trustworthy in the area of pacing. To the extent they had offloaded pacing responsibility to their devices, however, the runners didn't trust themselves either, leaving them in an untenable, rudderless state. Some resolved the dilemma by tuning out their device data altogether.

"I feel horrible when seeing that I am not keeping up with a pace that I planned," one runner said, "so I start thinking if I should push myself harder on the next kilometer or punish myself by running slow. . . . I just avoid looking at it at all and check once I'm done because it influences me in the wrong way. . . . It's just not that helpful, is it?" You couldn't ask for a better description of what it feels like when you just can't figure out how to transform running devices from a crutch, which is what they start off as for most runners, into the tool they must become for pacing mastery to be achieved.

Experience alone does not guarantee that a runner will eventually get to the point where they trust themselves more than their device. Not all of the experienced runners included in the Pierluigi Diotaiuti study described earlier escaped device overdependence. For that matter, most of the examples of device overdependence I shared above involved experienced athletes. Why do some runners escape device overdependence and master pacing while others struggle? What do they have that the rest lack?

In a word, *self-regulation*. A hot topic in the fields of sports psychology and general psychology, self-regulation is a general capacity, shared by all living organisms, to manage their internal states and behaviors according to the demands of a situation, and it is critical to pacing skill. As we will see in the next chapter, runners must either have or acquire a strong capacity to self-regulate to learn from experience and overcome device overdependence and the inherent difficulty of pacing to find their limit and run with confidence and control.

4

Pacing as Self-Regulation

Humans are not the only organisms that pace themselves during physical activity. Animals of all kinds depend for their survival on the ability to distribute their energy efficiently when engaging in life-or-death acts like hunting, escape, and migration. Take cheetahs, for example. Zoologists have observed that wild cheetahs run significantly farther in hunts that end in a successful kill than in hunts that don't. This suggests cheetahs are able to accurately judge whether they are likely to catch their prey, and when they deem success unlikely, they give up the chase in order to avoid wasting energy. Interestingly, the longest unsuccessful chases are usually carried out by young cheetahs, an indication that they do not yet know their limits as well as the more seasoned hunters do.

From a scientific perspective, pacing is classified as a form of self-regulation, defined by the editors of the *Handbook of Biobehavioral Approaches to Self-Regulation* as "a process that allows organisms to guide their behavior in pursuit of their goals." As such, self-regulation is fundamentally predictive in nature. Goals lie in the future. Pursuing them effectively therefore requires that the self-regulating organism be able to anticipate the future with a certain degree of accuracy. This is as true for human distance runners as it is for hunting cheetahs. In distance races, as we've seen, runners continuously assess their effort level in relation to the remaining distance and adjust their pace in the hope of crossing the finish line just as they reach their perceived limit. The crucial difference between this pacing task and a cheetah's hunting behavior is that the former requires the ability to comprehend abstract distances, which cheetahs lack. For better or worse, only humans can hunt invisible prey such as "10 kilometers" or "26.2 miles."

That which is uniquely possible for our species isn't necessarily easy for us, however. Much as young cheetahs struggle to know when a hunt is worth continuing and when to cut their losses, young and less experienced runners struggle to find their limit during competition. To date, most of the research tracking pacing skill development longitudinally has focused on types of endurance athletes other than runners, but we can be confident the findings apply to running. A 2015 study by British researchers found that 15-year-old competitive swimmers struggled to execute a basic pacing challenge (7 × 200 meters at incrementally increasing speeds), a failure that the authors attributed to both inexperience and cognitive immaturity. A separate study by German scientists reported that 17-year-old competitive swimmers performed much better in a comparable pacing challenge, indicating that 2 years of additional experience and maturation go a long way in adolescent swimmers aiming for pacing mastery.

Other research has shown that not all youth athletes improve equally in pacing skill over time. In 2017, the *International Journal of Sports Physiology and Performance* published the results of an ambitious 5-year effort led by Rikstje Wiersma and colleagues at the University of Groningen to track pacing skill development in a group of 104 youth speed skaters. Based on their recent competitive performances, the skaters were ranked initially as either elite, subelite, or nonelite. Interestingly, Wiersma's team found that, over the 5-year study period, skaters in all three categories evolved pacing patterns that looked more and more like those of world-class adult speed skaters, but the elite-level skaters showed significantly more improvement in this area than those of lower rankings.

What to make of these findings? I think we can safely assume that, in general, the young skaters who were classified as elite at the outset of the study were more physically talented than their lower-ranked peers. But what these results seem to suggest is that something else besides physical talent—something that enabled these athletes to gain pacing skill more quickly—was part of what made them elite in the first place.

In a 2017 article titled "Pacing and Self-Regulation: Important Skills for Talent Development in Endurance Sports," Marije Elferink-Gemser of the University of Groningen and Florentina Hettinga of Northumbria University offered the following answer to the question just posed:

> It seems that athletes who exhibit the greatest response to training, i.e., those who are most successful in improving their performance over time, are the ones who are eager to learn and train. They take responsibility for their own learning and training process, know which performance characteristics are important for them to develop, are highly motivated to improve and take action to do so. This goal-driven process is also described as self-regulation of learning and training, consisting of components of metacognition, motivation, and behavior. Self-regulation in general is the extent to which learners exert control over their own learning and training to master a specific task and to excel at it.

In other words, good learners make good pacers, and good self-regulators make good learners. The question then becomes, Where does a strong underlying capacity for self-regulation come from? If a runner needs to be adept at self-regulation not only to pace well today but also to learn to pace better tomorrow, what makes a runner (or any person) adept at self-regulation?

Psychologists have identified a number of mental traits that contribute to self-regulatory adeptness. Chief among them are body awareness, judgment, and toughness. There are others, but these three have the greatest relevance to the self-regulatory challenge of pacing a running event. Without exception, pacing masters are runners who possess all three traits to a high degree. Some are born with a head start and require little experience to develop their innate gifts of body awareness, judgment, and toughness to the level needed for pacing mastery. Others are less naturally gifted in one or more of these areas and must bootstrap their way toward having what it takes to become a pacing master.

In its dependence on fundamental mental traits, pacing is different from a lot of other skills, like knitting, that are not rooted in self-regulation. Whereas knitting ability is limited by manual dexterity and little else, pacing goes much deeper, drawing upon core features of our psychology. If you really want to become a pacing master, therefore, it might not be enough for you to gather experience and practice pacing exercises. These things are valuable, but so are the key mental aptitudes that support pacing skill, and unless you already possess these traits at the level of a Kenenisa Bekele, you stand to benefit from cultivating them.

Fear not—I haven't forgotten that I am a running coach, not a life coach. In this chapter and the next, I will focus narrowly on ways to cultivate body awareness, judgment, and toughness within the domain of running. I'll leave it to you to decide how interested you are in growing more broadly in these areas. Personally, I find it quite appealing that the journey toward pacing mastery goes as deep as you want it to. I mean, what an opportunity! Why merely improve as a runner when you can improve as a runner *and* become a better version of yourself in the process?

BODY AWARENESS

Can you feel your body right now? I'll bet you can. Every organism with a nervous system has the ability to feel its body in various ways. The scientific term for this ability is *interoception*. To function effectively in the world, we must not only feel our bodies but also know what we're feeling and act appropriately in response to what we feel. The hollow sensation we get when our stomach is empty, for example, must be correctly interpreted as a signal of hunger that prompts us to eat.

Beyond survival, interoception and related perceptions such as proprioception (awareness of the body in space) are vital to mastering a wide variety of skills. Body awareness in musicians is one example that has received special attention from scientists. A study involving guitarists found that years of practice had led to adaptations in the brain's structure and function that made the organ far more receptive to subtle nuances in afferent feedback from the fingers. We all have brains and fingers, but master guitarists have brains and fingers that can feel stuff ours can't. It's the same with running. Through training, runners get better at using specific forms of body awareness, including perception of effort, to aid their running.

Psychology research has demonstrated a strong link between interoceptive sensitivity (which is most often assessed by having subjects estimate their pulse rate by feel) and overall self-regulatory ability (which is measured through standardized inventories that ask subjects to rate their level of agreement with statements like, "If I make a resolution to change something, I pay a lot of attention to how I'm doing"). It makes sense, if you think about it. Interoceptive sensitivity requires that the mind be good at listening to the body, while self-regulation requires that the mind be good at talking to the body. It is only to be expected that the better the mind gets at listening to the body, the better it gets at telling it what to do, and vice versa.

Pacing, of course, is deeply dependent on the mind's ability to listen to and control the body. As body awareness goes up, therefore, so does pacing skill. But there are nuances to the process. Endurance training and competition do not increase body awareness in a simple, blanket fashion. Instead they lead to specific adaptations in body awareness that serve the runner's special interests. Take pain, for example. A 2020 study by Norwegian researchers compared pain processing in athletes (including distance runners) and nonathletes. Athletes were found to have a higher pain threshold (meaning higher levels of exposure to a painful stimulus were required before they registered pain) and a higher pain tolerance (meaning higher levels of a pain stimulus were required before they voluntarily withdrew from the stimulus) than nonathletes.

These results might seem to suggest that athletes have *less* body awareness than nonathletes, who are more sensitive and reactive to pain. But what they really indicate is a more adaptive relationship with pain, where the athlete has greater control of the perception. After breaking the men's world record for the marathon in Chicago, Kenya's Kelvin Kiptum was asked by a reporter if he had ever felt pain during any of his marathons. "I haven't," he said. This was an honest statement, I'm sure, yet I'm equally sure that if another person had felt what Kiptum was feeling in the final miles of his record-breaking performance, they would have called it pain. In any case, what's certain is that Kiptum's relationship with pain was a major reason he ran faster than any human ever had.

A pair of studies conducted by Welsh researchers and published in *PLOS One* in 2023 compared interoception in elite and nonelite runners and nonathletes. They found that runners exhibited more bodily trust and less body listening (or active attentional focus on body sensations) than nonathletes and that elite runners did even less body listening than nonelite runners. Like the pain study just described, these results suggest that endurance training and racing alter body awareness in ways that place the runner's mind in control, able to selectively tune out sensations that impede their goal pursuit and harness those that aid it.

The most illuminating experiments on body awareness in athletes are those demonstrating a direct connection between interoception and performance. An example is a 2011 study by researchers at the University of Lille involving 25 cyclists representing three levels of competitiveness: local, regional, and national. In the first part of the experiment, the cyclists were exposed to small doses of different exercise intensities and asked to estimate how long they could last at each. In the second part, the cyclists rode as long as they could at one of these intensities. All four of the locally competitive cyclists gave highly inaccurate predictions of their time to exhaustion, whereas four of the six national-caliber cyclists were spot-on in their estimates. The researchers concluded, "High-level athletes may be more consciously attuned to their bodies and their own effort sense as a result of greater exercise experience. They are more familiar with the signals of exertion emanating from acute cardiorespiratory, thermal and metabolic changes associated with an increase in exercise intensity than low-level athletes. Consequently, the task of interpreting these cues and using them to estimate their exhaustion time may be less prone to error and therefore may be less variable in this group."

There you have it. The goal of racing is to find one's limit, and the superior body awareness enjoyed by experienced and high-level athletes makes them better able to feel their way to their limit in competition. If an athlete's limit were fixed, mind you, this wouldn't matter much. They would have little need to adapt their pace to what they felt because their highest sustainable work rate would always be the same. In fact, though, the limit is ever-changing based on internal factors such as fitness and external conditions such as air temperature. Humans cannot run long distances as quickly in hot environments as in cool environments because doing so would cause the core body temperature to increase to dangerous levels. If we couldn't feel our bodies, we might try anyway, starting hot races at our normal speed and being forced to slow down or stop when we overheated. Thankfully, we can feel our bodies, so we instead reduce our pace very early in hot races, in reaction to sensed heat, when our core body temperature is still well below the danger zone. In fact, ingenious experiments involving radiant heat exposure have demonstrated that athletes pace themselves more conservatively even when it's just their skin that is warm and their core body temperature isn't affected at all.

A Master Class in Body-Aware Pacing

Not all runners have the level of body awareness needed to make the best pacing decisions. Even Olympians sometimes fail to make appropriate adjustments in adverse conditions. The 2004 Olympic Women's Marathon, for example, was held on a torrid summer evening in Athens, Greece. Despite a delayed start, the surface temperature was 95 degrees Fahrenheit when the racers bolted from the start line in Marathon, the ancient city that gave the event its name. Tucked away near the back of the throng was Deena Kastor of Team USA, heeding instructions she'd received from her husband, Andrew, 2 hours earlier in a cell phone call she'd placed to report on the conditions. "Just go slow," he'd said.

Not everyone did. The gold-medal favorite, Paula Radcliffe of Great Britain, surged to an early lead, trailing a retinue of sweat-soaked contenders unwilling to let the world record holder get away despite the punishing heat. Kastor, meanwhile, ran as though the others didn't exist, seeking shade wherever possible, drinking twice as much as she normally would, and holding a pace that, although markedly slower than she'd run in breaking the American marathon record in London the year before, was the fastest she felt she could sustain all the way to the Olympic Stadium in Athens. Whether or not it was fast enough to put her on the medal stand remained to be seen.

At 5 kilometers, Kastor was in 28th place, but the inevitable attrition began soon afterward, with runners who hadn't bothered to adjust cracking one by one. By 10 kilometers, Kastor had moved up to 17th place, and at the halfway point, only 11 runners remained in front of her. The only problem was that the leaders were *way* in front of her—nearly 2 minutes, and it seemed unlikely that 9 or more of those 11 would also crack, thereby opening the door for the pint-size Californian to snag a podium slot. But then Kenya's Margaret Okayo blew up, followed by her countrywoman Alice Chelangat, and then Radcliffe herself, who was seated on a curb, sobbing, when Kastor passed her 3.8 miles from the finish line. With less than a mile to go, a wobbling Elfenesh Alemu of Ethiopia ceded third place to Kastor, who powered home to claim the first Olympic marathon medal for an American woman since Joan Benoit won gold in Los Angeles in 1984.

Deena Kastor's performance in the 2004 Olympic Women's Marathon was a master class in pacing and an object lesson on the value of body awareness in the exercise of pacing skill. As it relates to running, this mental trait encompasses the full range of perceptions, beginning with the perception of effort, which, when properly attended to, can "tell" a runner how hard to push at any given moment of a race or workout. A runner who has a high level of body awareness *just knows* whether to speed up, slow down, or hold steady. Don't bother asking them to explain how. Body awareness, as it applies to pacing, is not unlike a singer's ability to match any pitch or an oenophile's ability to taste eight different flavors in a sip of wine. "Can't you hear that?" asks the singer. "Can't you taste that?" asks the wine connoisseur. And "Didn't you know that pace was too fast?" Deena Kastor might have asked the 25 runners who were ahead of her at the 5K point and behind her at the finish.

As I suggested in the preceding chapter, one of the reasons so many runners can't feel their bodies as well as the likes of Deena Kastor is that they don't grow up running, as she did. And I believe our 21st-century lifestyle also deserves some blame, its many comforts and conveniences having in a very real sense divorced our minds from our bodies. Such comforts and conveniences remain largely lacking in rural Kenya and Ethiopia, and this reality—the greater physicality of life in these places—may be yet another contributor to the success of the distance runners produced there.

So if you are not from these more active places, and you did not start running competitively in the sixth grade like Deena Kastor, how do you acquire the level of body attunement required to be a pacing master? I believe the most helpful things you can do are (1) make perceived effort your primary intensity metric in your training, at least for a while; (2) practice specific forms of mindfulness that are intended to enhance interoceptive sensitivity; and (3) perform certain types of runs that challenge body awareness. I will show you how to do all of these things in later chapters.

JUDGMENT

Pacing is, from one perspective, a series of decisions. Throughout each race, runners decide—sometimes consciously, other times at a gut level—to speed up, slow down, or maintain. A well-paced race, therefore, is the result of a lot of good decisions and few or no bad ones, which is another way of saying it is the result of good judgment. In this respect, running is far from unique among self-regulatory tasks. Remember, self-regulation is all about guiding one's behavior in pursuit of goals, and from weight loss to earning a law degree, it's hard to think of a goal that doesn't require making decisions.

Human decision-making has been studied since as far back as Plato, but increasingly scientists are approaching the subject from a self-regulatory perspective. Among the leading researchers in this area is Jacob Hirsh, a psychologist at the University of Toronto. In his PhD thesis, which was submitted and approved in 2010, Hirsh observed, "Pitting long-term goals against short-term desires is among the most difficult tasks in human decision-making." It is also precisely the kind of decision-making runners must do in races, where the long-term goal of getting to the finish line as quickly as possible is pitted against short-term desires that include not wanting to experience the discomfort that attends striving for one's limit. According to Hirsh, making these types of decisions involves a competition between "'hot' reward-focused impulses and 'cool' cognitive control mechanisms." The more successful the decision-maker is in overriding impulses when they are inconsistent with long-term goals, the more likely it is that a favorable outcome will be achieved.

To do their job effectively in these situations, the "cool" cognitive control mechanisms Hirsh refers to must be not only strong enough to override impulses but also keen enough to correctly judge when an impulse threatens to lead the decision-maker astray. In other words, the job of the "cool" system entails performance monitoring and error detection as well as decision-making and decision enforcement.

A brain area called the anterior cingulate cortex (ACC) is known to play an important role in these processes. Researchers commonly use an instrument known as the Stroop test to measure how well this part of the brain performs. Subjects are shown a series of individual words, all of which are names of primary colors, and each of which is presented in a primary-colored font. Sometimes the word and the font color match; other times they don't. The task of the test taker is to state the font color as quickly as possible, which is trickier than it sounds because one's instinct is to simply read the word. Performance is judged by the number of errors the subject makes and by how quickly answers are given. In research versions of the Stroop test, including Hirsh's, brain scans are conducted throughout the process. What these images reveal (among other things) is that when a subject realizes they have committed an error, the event is marked by an electrophysiological signal known as error-related negativity (ERN) in the ACC. The magnitude of the ERN is considered an indicator of the subject's ability to monitor their performance and to make performance-maximizing decisions, with larger magnitudes demonstrating greater ability in these areas.

As part of his thesis, Hirsh measured ERN magnitudes in a group of 31 college students as they completed a Stroop test. He then monitored the students' academic performance over the span of an entire school year, his expectation being that students with stronger cognitive control mechanisms, as evidenced by greater ERN magnitudes, would earn better grades. Hirsh explained his reasoning as follows: "Self-regulatory processes are thought to play an important role in the maintenance of academic goals. . . . Conceptually, this is because student GPA reflects the composite of many decisions made across a long period of time. For instance, a student has to decide on any given evening whether to study for a class or visit some friends. The result of each of these micro-decisions (each one a self-regulatory challenge) is reflected in ultimate academic performance. . . . Self-regulation reflects an improved ability to evaluate one's behaviour and engage the cool cognitive system whenever it is needed to sustain progress toward long-term goals." Sure enough, Hirsh found that students who exhibited stronger ERN signals during the Stroop test tended to get better grades.

The parallels between collegiate academic performance and running races are obvious. In much the same way a high GPA is the result of many small studying decisions, a well-executed race is the result of many small pacing decisions. We might therefore expect to see a link between Stroop test performance and running performance—and indeed we do. In 2015, the journal *PLOS One* published a study in which scientists at the University of Padua had 30 runners complete a pair of tests similar to the Stroop test that was designed to assess response inhibition or the ability of the cool cognitive control mechanisms to shut down hot reward-focused impulses. On the morning after these tests were completed, the runners participated in an 80 km ultramarathon, following which they were statistically separated into two groups: "faster runners" and "slower runners." Despite the fact that the decision-making tests were done at rest on a computer in street clothes and looked nothing at all like a running race, those who did well in one were found to have done better in the other also, evidence that better decision-making leads to better race execution.

The influence of judgment on pacing helps explain why female runners are generally better than male runners at pacing longer races, as was demonstrated in a 2021 study published in *Frontiers in Sports and Active Living*. Barry Smyth and Aonghus Lawlor at University College Dublin analyzed data from devices worn by more than 158,000 runners during a marathon and found that the average male runner lost 4.49 minutes compared to the average female runner as a result of starting too fast and losing steam. Other research has shown that men are generally more prone to risk-taking than women and that women's brains exhibit greater activity in the cool cognitive control centers of the brain when taking risks. Not all risks are the result of bad judgment, but aggressive starts to longer races are a bad judgment call that comes at a cost, to men especially. None of this means that male runners can't be as good as female runners at pacing longer races (as the example I'm about to share with you makes clear), but it does underscore the point that great pacing is impossible without good judgment.

What Good Pacing Judgment Looks Like

As I mentioned earlier, the mental trait we use to make good decisions is judgment. An example of what good judgment looks like when exercised in competition by a pacing master is Yuki Kawauchi's performance at the 2018 Boston Marathon. Yuki came to the race as a fan favorite but by no means a betting favorite to win. Nicknamed the "Citizen Runner," he worked a full-time job with the Japanese government and raced with legendary frequency. Indeed, he held the world record for the most sub-2:20 marathons run by a single athlete, but his PB of 2:08:14 was slower than those of defending champion Geoffrey Kirui (2:06:27) and several others in the field. Nevertheless, Yuki himself believed he could win if he played his cards right.

His plan was to go hard from the gun, a risky strategy that became even riskier when a nasty spring storm struck the Boston area on race morning. Despite facing a 25 mph headwind, Yuki went ahead with his gamble, running the first mile alone in 4:37. But his intent was not to lead the race from wire to wire. To have any chance of winning, Yuki knew he needed to make the race as hard as possible for everyone, so he was far from disappointed when the other contenders chased him down, engulfing the mismatched agitator (green vest, gray hat, red arm warmers, white gloves, orange shoes) at 5 km. Yuki then made a smart tactical shift, tucking in behind the taller Kirui and gathering his energy as he awaited the inevitable slowdown. When it came, he surged again, refusing to let his competitors get comfortable. A pattern formed: Over the next 20 kilometers, Yuki yo-yoed between brash pacemaking and cagey slipstreaming, doing just enough to keep his companions miserable. But Kirui had plans of his own, and when a whittled lead pack hit the hallowed hills of Newton, he revealed them, launching away so decisively that he was soon invisible, 90 seconds ahead of his nearest chaser.

Of the six runners caught flat-footed by the defending champion's attack, five had no choice in the matter—they were cooked. Only Yuki held back purposely, and it was his best decision in a day full of good decisions. Having scouted the second half of the racecourse on foot the day before (and the day before that), he felt Kirui's attack was too much too soon, and so he waited until he'd topped the dream-crushing Heartbreak Hill to give chase. By then, the defending champion was paying the price for his premature aggression. Yuki, half-blinded by fatigue and the elements, barely noticed passing the cratering Kenyan underneath the landmark Citgo sign en route to becoming the most unlikely Boston Marathon winner in recent memory.

Pundits credited Yuki's grit for his victory over faster rivals, but I believe his judgment was the decisive factor in this instance. Yuki had a smart plan, he was well prepared, and he executed his plan with the right mix of discipline and adaptability. There are five different modes in which judgment applies to pacing: planning, reactive tactical decisions, attentional focus, emotional self-regulation, and self-talk. Yuki handled all five of these modes masterfully before and during the 2018 Boston Marathon. Having set himself up for success by familiarizing himself with the course and committing to a fast start (planning), he ensured his success by pushing at the right times and not the wrong times (reactive tactical decisions), not getting discouraged when Kirui opened up a large lead (emotional self-regulation), ignoring everyone around him except the runners he judged most dangerous (attentional focus), and urging himself to finish with his best running in the final miles (self-talk).

Chances are you will never find yourself needing to practice good judgment in precisely the same ways Yuki did in order to win a future Boston Marathon, but you will need to handle the five modes of pacing-related decision-making with a similar degree of competence to achieve your best results, and I will show you how in the next chapter.

TOUGHNESS

The word *toughness* doesn't sound terribly scientific, but it is a recognized term in sports psychology. I find it interesting that every major running culture has a specific word for the same basic trait. In Finland they talk of *sisu*, which is usually translated as "spirit." The Ethiopian equivalent is *adegenna*, which means "dangerousness." Japanese runners strive for *ganbaru*, or "perseverance." And when American running legend Steve Prefontaine tossed around the word *guts*, his fellow anglophone runners knew exactly what he meant.

The many words for this one special quality that all great runners seem to possess tell us the phenomenon is both real and mysterious, definite yet difficult to define. Scholars of mental toughness agree. In a 2019 review paper, a group of authors led by Garry Kuan of Universiti Sains Malaysia observed, "Mental toughness appears to be multidimensional and most often associated with unshakable self-belief, the ability to rebound after failures (resilience), persistence or refusal to quit, coping effectively with adversity and pressure, and retaining concentration in the face of many potential distractions."

Sounds about right. But is mental toughness a single thing—as the umbrella term *toughness* suggests—or a bunch of related things, as suggested by the laundry list of qualities lumped together beneath this umbrella? The prevailing opinion among psychologists is that toughness is indeed a single, albeit multifaceted, thing. Among those who hold this view is Angela Duckworth, a researcher at the University of Pennsylvania who in 2016 coauthored a paper titled "Grit: Sustained Self-Regulation in the Service of Superordinate Goals." In it, Duckworth and her collaborators argue that toughness (or grit) is essentially everything other than motivation that enables and compels people to give everything they've got to complete a task or achieve a goal.

What I like about Duckworth's definition of toughness is that it's operational rather than conceptual, meaning it defines the phenomenon in terms of what it does and not by what it is. As such, it aligns with how the average person recognizes toughness. When we see a person persist in a challenge despite pain, suffering, hardship, fear, doubt, or long odds, we call it toughness, while Duckworth calls it sustained self-regulation in the service of superordinate goals, which is the same thing. This behavioral view of toughness puts an end to tedious debates about whether it is one thing or many and avoids the circularity of explaining a trait with other traits. Toughness is less a way of being than a way of doing, and any number of different traits may combine in a person to yield tough action.

Perfect race execution is a terrific example of a superordinate goal that requires self-regulation, hence toughness. To my knowledge, there is no existing scientific research demonstrating a direct connection between toughness and pacing skill, but there is plenty of indirect evidence. In ultramarathons, for example, failure to finish (referred to as "did not finish," or DNF) serves as a pretty good proxy for pacing skill—and for the toughness component of pacing skill, in particular. In a 2021 study, researchers at the University of Oviedo looked for correlations between various psychological variables and DNFs in a group of 356 participants in a mountain race. Of these runners, only 148 managed to complete the course. The strongest psychological predictors of a successful finish, according to the study's authors, were mental toughness and resilience (which overlaps with mental toughness). And not only that, but the toughest and most resilient runners among the nonquitters finished fastest.

Running is a painful sport, and as such, it selects for tough individuals who aren't afraid of a little suffering. But within the running population, some athletes are willing and able to suffer more than others, and only those who are willing to suffer the most realize their full potential in races. Remember, running performance is ultimately limited by perception of effort and not by fitness, which merely constrains performance.

A Lesson in Grit

The first half of the 2017 Run Rabbit Run 100-mile trail race was hard, but not harder than any other ultramarathon Courtney Dauwalter had done. She felt oddly out of sorts from the start, a feeling that wasn't helped by the 4,000-foot climb under a baking Colorado sun that served as the race's appetizer. Her husband Kevin's smile gave way to a look of concern as she stumbled into the first aid station at Mount Werner.

"I feel like I've run 70 miles already," she said.

She'd run 20 miles.

Shortly after leaving another aid station, Courtney threw up the entire contents of her stomach. *This is fine*, she thought (as she always did when it wasn't fine). In a sense, though, it was fine. There'd been rough patches in most of her prior ultras, including the previous year's edition of this very race, which she'd won. Sure enough, clouds rolled in as Courtney picked her way toward the aid station at Dry Lake, where she restocked her stomach with mashed potatoes and took the lead from Michelle Yates, and by 78 miles, she was feeling unstoppable, enjoying the playlist she'd prepared for the race and contemplating the course record.

That's when she noticed there was something wrong with her vision. It was half past two in the morning, and the temperature had dropped into the forties, so at first Courtney wondered if the haze she saw was fog, or perhaps her contact lenses were freezing. Only when she caught her toe on an unseen root and sprawled to the dirt did she acknowledge that the problem was internal and not helped by splashing water in her eyes.

She resumed running, spurred by the assumption that Lacy or another competitor was on her heels, and tumbled several times more as her sight worsened, the objects ahead smearing around the edges, the horizon flattening. She kept mum at the next aid station, letting people wonder about her bruises and grime-smeared clothes, but by the time she reached the final support stop back at Mount Werner, this was impossible. She'd smashed her forehead on a rock after tripping yet again and was bleeding copiously. By that point she'd gone completely blind, the pesky haze that first caught her attention intensifying to a perfect whiteout. Her world had collapsed to nothing, her shoes vanishing from sight beneath her, then her watch disappearing from her wrist (which had stopped in an earlier fall, so no matter). Upon rising from the dirt and feeling liquid dripping down the left side of her face, she wiped her fingers across her forehead and inspected them for blood, but even with her palm held right in front of her nose, she couldn't tell.

At no point did Courtney consider stopping or even reducing her pace from a run to a walk. Nor was she alarmed at the strangeness of her sudden blindness. To her it was just the latest challenge, categorically equal to more common ultramarathon challenges like sore legs and puking. One of the hallmark characteristics of toughness is a kind of stoical indifference to difficulties of all kinds. It's not that tough people don't suffer. They just don't care. All roads are the same to them. Whether smooth or rocky, up or down, they lead to the destination, which is all that matters.

As she bombed her way down the single-track Mountain View Trail (having chucked one of her contacts to test whether she'd see better without it—she didn't), Courtney encountered a series of runners in the 50-mile division making their way toward her. Although she couldn't see them, she heard their cries of alarm. *Whoa! Are you okay?* The humor of her predicament wasn't lost on Courtney. *At least I'm making their day a little more interesting*, she thought. She smiled at the mental image of a brown bear pausing its breakfast as she lurched past and wondering, *What the hell was that?*

"I have a little bit of a problem," she confessed to the volunteers at Mount Werner.

Unable to persuade Courtney to quit, the aid station captain radioed race director Paul Sachs and got his permission to send a guide with Courtney for the remaining 6 miles. Pacers are not permitted at Run Rabbit Run, so the guide ran behind her, calling out warnings like "Sharp right turn ahead!" and "It's about to get a little steeper!" The last section of the course along the Storm Peak Challenge Trail was undulating. Powerless to anticipate its rises and dips, Courtney plowed into the former like a barge on high seas and felt her stomach flip like a roller coaster rider when the trail dropped out from underneath her feet.

The finish line was marked by a giant red balloon sculpture. Courtney ran unseeing straight through it and into the arms of Paul Sachs, who for all she knew was "just some random creeper," as she joked in a later interview. Her vision returned gradually over the next several hours.

Performances like this one are deeply inspiring because they show us what is possible with a strong mind. At the same time, they are somewhat intimidating—because they show us what is possible with a strong mind! "What's your excuse?" they seem to ask. To watch a Courtney Dauwalter compete is to be forced to admit that we have not yet found our limit in the toughness department. No runner can claim to have paced a race optimally unless they have left absolutely everything they had to give out on the course, and runners like Courtney are only too happy to remind us of this fact.

What does it take to give it 100 percent? I'll answer this question by asking another: Do you remember the lesson of *The Wizard of Oz*? In giving the Scarecrow a diploma, the Tin Man a testimonial, and the Cowardly Lion a medal of courage, the Wizard pointed out that only a person who had a brain would want a brain, and that only a person who had a heart would want a heart, and, yes, that only a person who had courage (or toughness) would want it. If, as a runner, you earnestly desire to become tougher, you're already halfway there. The rest is just details. As American record holder Ryan Hall said, "The best way to become a mentally tough runner is to believe that you're a mentally tough runner."

There's much more to be said about the mind of the pacing master, where toughness combines so fruitfully with body awareness and judgment. Let's have a look inside.

5

The Mind of a Pacing Master

The best pacer I've ever run with is Ben Bruce, a now retired professional runner and former member of the Flagstaff-based HOKA Northern Arizona Elite team. When I joined the group as an honorary member in the summer of 2017, I was far too slow to do anything other than easy runs with Ben and his fellow elites, but as luck would have it, Ben was injured that summer, and he was kind enough to pace me through a few key sessions while rehabbing what, at the time, he thought was a hip flexor strain but turned out to be a pelvic stress fracture.

The first of these sessions was a long progression run on Lake Mary Road, a hallowed proving ground for Flagstaff-based marathoners. As Ben ran alongside me, I was struck not only by his ability to nail the mile splits I gave him but also by how much thought he put into the process. Aware that I would be doing a lot more running, most of it alone, on the same highway in the coming weeks, Ben shared a litany of tips on how to stay on pace, noting tricky false flats, exposed stretches where headwinds were common, sharp descents that offered opportunities to bank time, and so forth.

In light of this experience, I wasn't the least bit surprised when Ben later transitioned into a coaching role with NAZ Elite that involved extensive pacing work. His pièce de résistance was a job leading Keira D'Amato to the seventh-fastest marathon time ever recorded by an American woman (2:22:56) at the 2020 Marathon Project in Chandler, Arizona. It was, I'll grant, a relatively straightforward pacing task, given the course's pancake-flat, multiloop layout, which facilitated a steady rhythm, but Ben made it look much easier than it was, shepherding Keira through 5 km splits of 17:02, 16:58, 17:02, 16:59, 16:55, 16:59, 16:55, and 16:56 before Keira dropped the hammer over the last 2.2 km as Ben peeled off.

If you're skeptical of the notion that some runners have an innate knack for pacing, good luck explaining Ben Bruce's mastery. Raised in San Diego, he got a relatively late start as a running specialist, competing in his first-ever track race as a college freshman after earning varsity letters in golf, soccer, and cross country during his high school years. Yet despite having less experience than his fellow Cal Poly Mustangs, Ben was by far the most reliable pacer on the team. In acknowledgment of this, the senior captains awarded him the pressure-laden honor of leading the crucial first repetition in workouts.

In Chapter 8, we'll talk about macropacing, or pacing on a long time scale. Many if not most runners who are good at pacing individual runs are equally good at pacing their overall running career. Ben proved to be great at both, pacing himself to a professional running career that lasted nearly 2 decades, earning the distinction of being the only runner ever to qualify for and compete in 16 straight USATF Outdoor Championships. And though he might not like my mentioning it, Ben is also the only runner ever to have finished 10th, 9th, 8th, 7th, 6th, 5th, 4th, 3rd, and 2nd—but never 1st—in national championship races.

The secret to Ben's pacing mastery is no secret. Like all pacing masters, Ben is a virtuosic self-regulator on the roads, trails, and track, endowed with all three of the key mental traits that pacing skill depends on. Body awareness? Check. Ben showed exceptional interoceptive at the 2023 Big Sur Marathon, which he started on tired legs, having raced the Boston Marathon just 6 days before. Battling vicious headwinds gusting up to 35 miles per hour (not to mention 2,192 feet of climbing), Ben tuned his effort perfectly to the unique conditions, finishing 46 seconds ahead of the fast-closing second-place runner with his last drop of energy. Judgment? Also check. Ben's remarkable judgment was expressed in a patient, methodical, even-keeled approach to training and development that enabled him to just keep getting better and better year after year. "I have always had a consistent mindset," he said in a 2012 interview for RunCoach.com. "Chipping away at times over the years has been the way that I have gotten to where I am as a runner today. . . . Not any one workout will make you a superstar, but a bunch of solid ones will make you super strong and ready to race." Toughness?

Checkmate! I saw Ben's toughness firsthand in the summer of 2017, when he ran through the pain of an as-yet undiagnosed pelvic stress fracture that would have immobilized most runners.

As a coach, Ben shares my belief that you don't have to be a natural-born pacing master like him to become one. The preceding chapters served to define the mission: To master the skill of pacing, one must cultivate the capacity to self-regulate both during runs (exercising behavioral control in relation to the goal of finding one's limit) and between runs (exercising behavioral control in relation to the goal of learning to pace better). Cultivating the capacity to self-regulate, in turn, requires the development of body awareness, judgment, and toughness. The goal of this chapter is to offer practical instruction on how to do this. None of the methods you'll learn here qualifies as a quick fix, much less a "hack." The road to pacing mastery is long, but there's a prize at the end of it—the sublime joy of running free, which is to say, of knowing what you can do and then going out and doing it every time.

LEARNING BODY AWARENESS

A distinction can be made between general body awareness and task-specific body awareness. General body awareness, or interoceptive sensitivity, is the broad capacity to feel one's body, which is measured through tests such as counting one's heartbeats by feel. Specific body awareness is the trained feel for certain body parts or movements that comes through skill development. The task-specific body awareness that, for example, a tightrope walker develops through training for his vocation is different from the body awareness that a runner develops through training for her sport. Whereas the tightrope walker learns a refined sense of balance, the runner hones a precise perception of effort as well as other kinds of interoceptive sensitivity, including the kind Kenenisa Bekele used to keep his hamstring from shredding while fighting to remain in contention for victory in the 2019 Berlin Marathon.

As a runner, you're not interested in developing forms of body awareness that have little relevance to your sport. The time and energy you invest in improving your body awareness need to go toward measures that offer the greatest benefit to your running. Three of my favorites are body scanning, condition assessment, and time-limit estimation.

Body Scanning

Research has demonstrated that meditation and other forms of mindfulness (a state of receptive attention to the present moment) improve body awareness by modulating the insula, a brain region involved in interoception. Body scanning is a mindfulness practice that targets body awareness directly, and it can be done both during running and at rest.

RUNNING BODY SCAN

To scan your body while running, focus your attention on one small piece of your overall experience at a time, pausing long enough to notice everything there is to notice before moving on to the next piece. Your breathing is a good place to start. Don't try to control or change it; just notice it. Take some time to attend to your perception of effort. Try to pick up its nuances. Words such as *hard* and *easy* don't even begin to capture all that's going on with effort perception at any given moment. For example, the sort of hard effort you might experience when running slowly in a state of extreme fatigue is very different from the sort you might experience during the third lap of a 1-mile track race.

Other aspects of the running experience you can focus on include soreness and other forms of discomfort in your musculoskeletal system, the rhythm of your arm and leg movements, specific parts of your body (even your toes!), the tension in your face and shoulders, your perception of speed and movement through space, and the various interfaces between your body and the environment: contact between your feet and the ground, gravitational resistance, and the feeling of air brushing against your skin.

Runners are always aware of their bodies when running, of course, but conducting a formal body scan while running is as different from this default awareness as meditation is from daydreaming. The goal is not to scan your body continuously throughout every run—that would drive you nuts. Focusing too much on internal perceptions is actually harmful to performance, for reasons I will explain when we explore race pacing in Chapter 7. Just scan your body for a few minutes at a time when it crosses your mind to do so. Over time, you will develop a better sense of how to interpret and use what you're feeling to inform your pacing decisions.

BODY SCAN MEDITATION

If you practice meditation, adding body scan meditations to your routine can be a nice complement to running body scans. These can be done anytime—before a run, after a run, or whenever you normally meditate. Sit comfortably in a quiet environment and allow your attention to roam from one focal point to the next. Start by attending to the overall position of your body, then concentrate on where you are in space and how you're feeling generally (e.g., warm, calm, thirsty). Next, seek out areas of tension in your body, just noticing the feeling rather than trying to get rid of it, and then shift to your breathing. Now move your attention slowly from the top of your head to your face, neck, shoulders, chest and heart, arms, torso, stomach, bottom, upper legs, knees, lower legs, ankles, feet, and toes. Finally, do the whole thing in reverse, returning step by step to the overall position of your body.

If you're so inclined, include a heart rate estimation test in the occasional body scan meditation. To do this, you will need to wear a heart rate monitor with a timer. Take a few moments to focus your attention on the feeling of your heart muscle's contractions. Start the timer and begin to count the contractions. Continue for 1 minute, then stop the time and check your total against the current heart rate reading on your watch. See if you can improve your accuracy with repeated practice. You can be sure that any improvement you do achieve will translate into better interoceptive sensitivity when running, hence better pacing ability.

Condition Assessment

When I last spoke to Ben Bruce, I asked him how fast he thought he could run a 10K race at his present fitness level. Without hesitation, he answered, "Twenty-nine something." Mind you, Ben wasn't training for a 10K at the time. His recent running had lacked any real structure, consisting of a mix of pacing work for NAZ Elite members and easy runs done on a catch-as-catch-can basis. Yet he seemed quite confident in his prediction, and I have no doubt that his answer would have proved accurate had he given in to my arm-twisting and actually raced a 10K the next day.

Where does this kind of self-knowledge come from? I believe it comes largely from condition assessment, a practice whereby runners use each and every run they do to assess their present fitness level. This is something all runners—including those who struggle with pacing—do when circumstances demand it, such as when a runner who is training for a 10K race does a set of intervals targeting a 10K race pace. But pacing masters like Ben conduct a form of condition assessment in all their runs, and the sheer volume of information generated through this habit is what makes the difference. Put another way, what makes a pacing master a pacing master is that they get a feel for how fast they could race a 10K not just from a 10K-pace workout performed on relatively fresh legs but also from a random, short recovery run performed on tired legs the day after a hard workout.

To succeed in gleaning information about your fitness level from runs of various kinds, you must properly contextualize what you're feeling. Let's return to the example of a run that comes the day after a hard workout. It's likely, of course, that you will feel tired and run slow in any such run. But it's possible that you will feel somewhat less tired and go somewhat faster than you have in recent runs performed in similar circumstances, and if you do, you may conclude from this information that your training is going well and you're getting fitter.

When conducting condition assessments, it's helpful to place today's run in an even broader context, comparing how you're feeling and performing—all things considered—against how you've felt and performed in similar circumstances in previous training cycles. Again, one such comparison won't tell you much, but routine comparisons of this type will aid you in setting goals and performance expectations for upcoming races.

Just be careful not to allow your condition assessments to become a source of anxiety. Approached with the wrong mindset, this practice could easily cause you to train in a state of perpetual worry about whether you are on track toward a goal, sort of like how weighing yourself too often or obsessively checking your stock portfolio can make you freak out needlessly. It's a matter of keeping perspective. If you complete a long run on a hot day after a poor night's sleep with 13 weeks remaining before a marathon, when you're still relatively far from peak fitness, don't interpret the misery you experience in the late miles as proof that you're doomed to fail in your marathon. Conduct your condition assessments with a mindset of neutral curiosity. Account for everything—the heat, the lack of sleep, your modest fitness level, the 13 weeks you've got to get fully race-ready—in assessing your condition, and maintain the same neutral mindset in all of your condition assessments. Don't interpret your runs as if your race is tomorrow unless, in fact, your race is tomorrow.

Time-Limit Estimation

Another simple exercise that you can perform routinely in the course of your normal training is time-limit estimation. This practice entails asking yourself how long you think you could sustain your present pace or, alternatively, selecting a pace you feel you could sustain for a specific amount of time. Like condition assessments, time-limit estimation, when used intentionally as a tool for learning body awareness, is nothing more than a broadened application of something all runners do automatically in races and time trials, during which every runner estimates, consciously or unconsciously, how long they can keep up their current pace.

Experience supplies runners with a general idea of how long it's going to take to complete a run, and at each point along the way, we ask ourselves, explicitly or implicitly, *Can I hold this pace the rest of the way?* Experiments like the University of Lille study mentioned in Chapter 4 have shown that higher-performing endurance athletes are better at estimating how long they can sustain a given output, and that's why conscious time-limit estimation is a worthwhile pacing exercise.

Like condition assessments (and body scanning), this exercise is one you can sprinkle into your training in a playful way, employing it whenever the mood strikes you. Again, we're all accustomed to estimating our time limit in races and time trials, but what I'm advocating is conscious use of the same faculty in other situations—easy runs, long runs, tempo runs, whenever. It's just another way of making you more mindful of what your body's telling you about its abilities and limits.

Time-limit estimation is also useful as a way to regulate intensity in runs. Such estimates may either replace or supplement objective metrics used for the same purpose, such as pace. For example, most runners, regardless of fitness or ability, are able to sustain their VO_2max pace (or the slowest pace at which they achieve their maximal rate of oxygen consumption) for about 6 minutes. Therefore, you can target VO_2max intensity in an interval workout by selecting a pace you feel you could sustain for 6 minutes.

Even when you do choose to use an objective measure as your primary intensity metric in a given run, estimated time limits have a role to play, helping you find the appropriate effort quickly before your device has a chance to catch up to a shift in speed and also helping you adjust your pace as you go based on factors like elevation change and fatigue. I'll have more to say on this subject in the next chapter.

CULTIVATING JUDGMENT

Similar to body awareness, judgment operates on two levels: general and task specific. At both levels, judgment expresses itself through decisions. People who have general good judgment make good decisions in most areas of their lives. But we all know people who make good decisions within a special area of expertise while showing poor judgment in other areas. Every great athlete makes consistently good decisions within their sport, but not every great athlete also makes good decisions with money, in relationships, and elsewhere. To master the skill of pacing, you will need to cultivate better pacing judgment, and the way to do it is reasonably straightforward.

Research has shown that teaching athletes sport-specific decision-making skills improves their judgment on the field of play. A 2013 study conducted by Spanish researchers and published in *PLOS One* explored the effect of decision-making skills training on junior tennis players. Eleven players were separated into two groups, both of which played 18 full matches that were videotaped. The first four matches were used to establish a baseline (so to speak) of decision-making competence.

After each of the next 10 matches, the 5 members of the decision-making skills training group sat down to review a tape of selected points with a coach, who asked the players to explain and critically evaluate their decisions in a guided manner. The six members of the control group received no such training. In the last four matches, decision-making competence was reassessed. On average, players in the decision-making skills training group were found to have improved their decision-making scores by 10 percent, whereas the players in the control group showed no improvement.

In my one-on-one work with runners, I've found that a similarly intentional approach to improving decision-making can improve pacing judgment. The tool I rely on most for this purpose is decision tracking, which is similar to the method used in the study just described. The key difference is that there's no video involved. It's just a mental performance review that can be done in the context of your training log. After each workout or run involving important pacing decisions, devote some space in your training log to assessing your decisions in the five areas that I first enumerated in Chapter 4: planning, emotional self-regulation, self-talk, tactical adjustments, and attentional focus.

Planning

Pacing decisions are made before a run even begins. This goes for both races and training runs, but for now, let's focus on training. Among the decisions you'll need to put some thought into before training runs are where to run, what your pace and time targets will be, and who to run with. There's no need to fuss over such decisions ahead of less important workouts, but when there's a lot riding on a particular run, you'll want to set yourself up for success in every way possible (for example, find someone like Ben Bruce to run with you!).

The most common mistake runners make in setting workout pace targets is basing their decisions on their aspirations rather than on a realistic assessment of their current fitness. Aspirational workout goals inevitably lead to overreaching and frustration. Remember to always train as the athlete you are today, not as the athlete you hope to be on race day. Ensuring that your training consistently meets you where you are is precisely how you become the athlete you hope to be down the road.

Be sure to give yourself credit for good decisions as readily as you call yourself out for bad decisions. The researchers who conducted the tennis experiment I just described made a point (so to speak) of having subjects review as many situations in which they made the right decision as those in which they chose the wrong move. So, for example, if procrastination left you with no option other than to run in the heat of the afternoon, thereby putting out of reach a target pace that would have been manageable in the cool of the morning if you'd only gotten your lazy ass out of bed, take yourself to task. And if you nail a workout after turning down an invitation from a friend who always half-steps you and drags you out of your proper rhythm, pat yourself on the back. In either case, the process will improve future decisions.

Emotional Self-Regulation

Affect, or emotion, plays an important and underappreciated role in pacing. Remember, pacing is the art of finding your limit, and negative thoughts and feelings make it harder—impossible, really—to reach your true limit. This was shown in a fascinating study conducted by researchers at the University of Worcester and published in the *International Journal of Sports Physiology and Performance*. Fourteen runners completed 10K performance tests on two occasions—once alone and once in a group. On average, they ran 58 seconds faster in the group test, yet their pacing patterns were the same in both. The difference was that the runners experienced higher levels of positive affect in the group 10K. In other words, they ran closer to their limit with others because they were enjoying themselves more.

You, too, will perform better if you keep your emotions within the neutral-to-positive range and out of the negative zone in races and workouts. One way to do this is with positive self-talk, which is the subject of the next section. But before you can engage in positive self-talk, you sometimes need to stop negative thoughts. This entails mentally "catching" negative thoughts quickly and overriding them. For example, you might start thinking "I hate how I'm feeling right now" during a workout, then realize you're thinking this and consciously put a stop to it. Doing so won't change the fact that you're suffering, but it will keep your mind from exacerbating the situation and dragging down your performance.

Acceptance is another technique that is proven to mitigate negative thoughts and feelings during exercise and thereby enhance performance. This entails making peace or being okay with your discomfort. You're not trying to persuade yourself that you're not really uncomfortable—that doesn't work. Rather, you're accepting your discomfort as a necessary part of the task you're performing. You can't control how you feel when you're running, but you can control how you feel about how you feel, and acceptance is the most performance-enhancing feeling you can possibly have about exertional discomfort. Research has shown that consciously accepting discomfort increases endurance performance. It's mainly a matter of embracing the fact that discomfort is inextricably linked to the things that make finding your limit worthwhile for you. As the Nepalese elite ultrarunner (and former adolescent guerrilla fighter) Mira Rai said in an interview for the *Mindful Running* podcast, "Running makes me happy. When you're happy doing whatever you do, pain becomes secondary."

Acceptance works best when it begins before running. You accept that the run is going to hurt, and then, when it does, you accept that it does, which is always easier to do when the discomfort is anticipated. In a 2021 interview for *Athletics Weekly*, Norwegian elite middle-distance runner Jakob Ingebrigtsen described how he uses this anticipatory acceptance technique in racing:

> I usually get really nervous, not only because of my expectations but it's also about the pain. . . . I don't enjoy being in pain. . . . If you are really well prepared and you do what you need to do going into that race, it's going to end up pretty good, and you're not going to feel that much pain after all. But I know, going into my next race, I get really nervous [again] because of the pain. But I think that's my way of preparing myself physically and mentally for each race—to be nervous of the pain that's coming but also to be awake and focused on the task so I can run as fast as possible.

It's worth mentioning that Ingebrigtsen was only 20 years old when he spoke these words. You can be certain he wouldn't have accomplished all he had at such a young age (having already set numerous national and European records and won European and World Championships medals, he's gone on to win three Olympic and World Championship gold medals) without such a strong capacity for emotional self-regulation. Take a cue from Jakob Ingebrigtsen and, as part of your postrun decision tracking, rate how well you regulated your emotions before and during it. Give yourself full credit for successful thought stopping and acceptance, and admit where you fell short.

Self-Talk

I've always thought of "self-talk" as being a little corny. It brings to mind children's stories like *The Little Engine That Could* or Al Franken's Stuart Smalley sketch on *Saturday Night Live*—"I'm good enough, I'm smart enough, and doggone it, people like me!" Corny or not, though, self-talk impacts pacing, for better or worse. The kind of encouragement these fictional characters gave themselves is proven to enhance endurance performance. A study led by Samuele Marcora and published in *Medicine & Science in Sports & Exercise* in 2014 reported that training in positive self-talk improved performance in a high-intensity ride to exhaustion by 17 percent.

This type of "note to self" works best if it has personal significance or addresses a specific need. One-size-fits-all mantras like "I think I can" are better than nothing, but you'll get more mileage out of phrases that speak to your individual weaknesses and immediate challenges. For example, if you are prone to self-doubt, and you find such feelings bubbling up at a tough moment in a race or workout, you might choose to think, "Nothing to prove," to remind yourself that you are worthy, win or lose, and all that matters is trying your best. And if you find yourself beginning to overheat during a race and are concerned that dialing back your effort in response to this feeling will put your podium ambitions in jeopardy, you might choose to think, "It's hot for everyone, not just me."

Self-talk can also be used in more tactical ways to assist pacing. Two-time Olympian and world champion Ajeé Wilson of the United States liked to mentally divide her 800-meter races into two parts: the first 300 meters, which were all about positioning herself for the last 500 meters, and those painful last 500 meters, at the start of which she mentally recited the same script every time: *You're okay. You're comfortable. You're fine.*

Does every great half-miler use this same script? In other words, is Wilson's self-talk ritual necessary to optimize pacing in an 800-meter race? It is not. But tactical self-reminders of some kind, which can vary from runner to runner and from event to event, *are* required to find your limit, and they are equally helpful in workouts that run below the limit. Over time, decision tracking can help you discover the particular internal messages that work best for you, just like Ajeé Wilson.

Tactical Adjustments

When Ben Bruce set his half-marathon personal best in Tempe, Arizona, in 2016, he faced a critical decision around 5 miles, where the lead pack he'd been running in broke apart as top contenders Scott Bauhs and Karim El Mabchour accelerated to a pace that felt a bit too quick for Ben. There were two options: go with the pacesetters anyway and risk hitting the wall or avoid this risk by holding back and giving up on any chance of winning. He opted to roll the dice, and at 10 miles, he found himself not only still in contention but feeling surprisingly strong, so he continued to press, chasing Bauhs all the way to the finish line for second place.

This is one example of the sort of tactical pacing decision runners are required to make all the time in workouts and, especially, in races. Over the course of a longer event like a half-marathon, dozens of such decisions are made, and they range from slowing down and tucking behind a taller athlete while running into a headwind to disregarding a mile split that's so far off expectations as to suggest the possibility of measurement error.

It is beyond the scope of this book to offer comprehensive guidance on how to handle every conceivable type of tactical pacing decision you might encounter. Nor should you want such guidance. The goal is to become confident in your own ability to handle tactical decisions, not to have these decisions made for you!

In all seriousness, the tactical element of pacing is one of those things that's more learnable than teachable. By this I mean that intentional practice will take you a lot further than an encyclopedia of if-then instructions from me or any coach. For this reason, decision tracking is especially valuable in its application to tactical pacing decisions. It doesn't matter how bad your tactical decision-making is today. By reviewing and grading your pacing decisions routinely, you will become increasingly confident in the calls you make in the heat of the moment. But what if you lack the confidence to even distinguish good pacing decisions from bad ones? In this case, consider working with a coach to build a base of knowledge for your confidence to rest on.

Attentional Focus

The relevance of attentional focus to pacing is obvious. No runner has ever paced a race or hard workout optimally by daydreaming their way through it—at least not that I'm aware of.

There's an almost infinite variety of things you can focus your attention on when running, but all fall within a handful of broad categories. At the most general level, your attention can be focused either externally or internally. When focused externally, your attention can be directed toward task-relevant stimuli, such as a big puddle on the trail ahead that you'll want to avoid splashing through, or non-task-relevant stimuli, such as a squirrel scampering across a tree branch above you.

When focused inward, your attention may be directed toward thoughts, emotions, body sensations, physiological processes including breathing, and actions such as your step rate. These too may be either task relevant (an example being assessing your thirst intensity) or non–task relevant (like wondering how the Green Bay Packers are doing in their big showdown against the Chicago Bears). An internal attentional focus may also be metacognitive, meaning you're thinking about what you're thinking or feeling, an example of which is assessing whether your current perceived effort level is appropriate for the moment.

All of these examples of attentional focus may also be proactive or reactive in nature. Proactive attention entails choosing its object, as when you glance at your device to check the elapsed time, while reactive attention entails responding to a stimulus, often involuntarily, as when you hear your name shouted and glance to the right, where you see your cousin Sam cheering you on.

Research has shown that certain uses of attentional focus tend to aid performance, while others tend to hinder it. Broadly speaking, non-task-relevant foci like thinking about what you're going to eat after the race are unhelpful. Sometimes you'll hear disappointed elite runners chastise themselves in post-race interviews for "losing focus." Seldom are such lapses as egregious as making mental shopping lists during competition, but virtually any distraction from the task at hand will negatively affect pacing and performance.

The mental trick known as chunking can be helpful in maintaining focus during longer events, where staying focused is especially challenging. Sports psychologist Noel Brick, whose research concentrates on how elite endurance athletes use their minds during training and competition, defines this trick as "mentally breaking down the distance to smaller segments." Thirty kilometers into a 50K ultramarathon, thinking about the finish line may be overwhelming, but thinking about reaching the next aid station is far less so.

The one circumstance in which dissociation, or intentionally not focusing on the task at hand, can be beneficial is when a runner's discomfort level verges on intolerable. There's a great example of helpful dissociation in novelist Haruki Murakami's memoir, *What I Talk About When I Talk About Running*. While competing in his first ultramarathon, Murakami hit a rough patch during which he tried every psychological trick he could think of to keep running despite the overpowering desire he felt to stop. As a last-ditch measure, he tried telling himself, "I'm not a human. I'm a piece of machinery. I don't need to feel a thing. I just forge on ahead." To his amazement, this self-admittedly unhinged internal pep talk worked. Murakami did not literally turn into a machine, of course, nor did he actually cease to feel a thing, but somehow the very repetition of this thought enabled him to find a certain peace within his suffering and catch a second wind. "My muscles silently accepted this exhaustion now as a historical inevitability, an ineluctable outcome of the revolution," he writes. "I had been transformed into a being on autopilot, whose sole purpose was to rhythmically swing his arms back and forth, move his legs forward one step at a time." In this trancelike state, Murakami found himself easily passing the scores of runners who had passed him during his earlier rough patch. "It's weird, but at the end I hardly knew who I was or what I was doing," he reflects. "By then running had entered the realm of the metaphysical. First there came the action of running, and accompanying it there was this entity known as me. I run; therefore I am."

As I say, though, except in emergencies, dissociation tends to harm pacing and performance, as does thinking about or trying to control physiological processes such as breathing. Focusing on your movements can go either way. As a general rule, doing so is helpful when your attention is directed toward the interface between your body and the environment or on staying relaxed, whereas it's unhelpful when it's used to try to run "correctly" in some way. In a study that Noel Brick did on mental processes in elite runners during training and racing, self-reminders to relax were among the most commonly cited metacognitive strategies.

Different situations demand different attentional foci, and studies involving elite endurance athletes indicate that the highest performers are adept at selecting the right focus for each moment. If you think about it, this makes sense. In the early part of a marathon, for example, when you're feeling energized and excited, it might be best to pay extra attention to the current pace reading on your device as a way to prevent overzealous pacing, whereas in the late part of a marathon, it's better to ignore your device completely in favor of feeling your way to the limit and urging yourself forward with positive self-talk.

TABLE 5.1. The do's and don'ts of attentional focus in runs

DO	DON'T
Think helpful thoughts	Allow negative thoughts and emotions to go unchecked
Stay focused on task-relevant stimuli	Dissociate
Allow your main focus to be context specific	Think about your breathing or other automated physiological processes
Relax	
	Try to control your form
Let your attention roam among a few key foci	Fixate on one thing

At all times, though, your attention should roam. Whether you're 2000 meters into a 10,000-meter track race or working your way through hill repetition number 6 in a set of 10, you'll get the best outcome if you shift your attention from one object to another within a limited set of perceptions, thoughts, and emotions. Pacing masters develop a natural rhythm in their attention cycling, a sort of attentional loop that moves from effort assessment to context-specific self-talk to pace checking and back to effort assessment (for example), with allowances for reacting to salient stimuli and changing the contents of the loop as the run unfolds.

The opposite of such tactical attentional roaming is fixation. Allowing your mind to fixate on something is almost always harmful to pacing and performance. Most often this occurs when a runner is experiencing a high level of discomfort, which then dominates their attention in the way that extreme pain does, but there are also many examples of runners fixating on less threatening elements of their experience such as negative thoughts ("I'm behind my goal pace") or emotions (such as disappointment) or even device data. At a press conference I attended after the 2010 Boston Marathon, a reporter asked Ryan Hall why he'd looked at his watch so frequently during the first mile of the race, which Hall had completed in 4:36. Hall explained that he had done it in an effort to keep himself in check, having run the same mile in an absurdly quick 4:29 in his Boston debut 2 years earlier. Not quite satisfied with this answer, the reporter informed Hall that he'd glanced at his watch no fewer than 17 times in that first mile.

"I guess that is a bit excessive," Hall laughed.

So, hey, even the pros do it. But just as Ryan Hall (who, by the way, finished third that day in 2:08:40) admitted to fixating too much on his watch in the opening mile of the 2010 Boston Marathon, you, too, should confess your errors in attentional focus in your training log while also noting what you did right. Table 5.1 presents the basic dos and don'ts of attentional focus during running, which you can use in making these assessments. Note that they apply only in races and workouts where your goal is to find or approach your limit. Different rules apply in easy runs, which we will talk about in the next chapter.

BUILDING TOUGHNESS

I am living proof that a runner doesn't have to be born tough to become tough. As a high school runner, my aversion to the pain of racing was so extreme that I committed unforgivable acts of cowardice such as faking injuries to escape it. When I got back into competitive running in my late twenties—having quit years before to escape the pain of racing once and for all—I was determined to exorcise the demons that sabotaged the first act of my running life, which meant embracing the suffering I'd previously shied away from. In this second act of my running life, the pain of racing was no longer just a vitiating part of the experience but the very point of it. I wanted not just to run well but to see myself as a tough person, and to this end, I measured myself less by how quickly I ran than by how close I got to my absolute limit in the effort to run quickly.

Success didn't come overnight, but it did come. I will never forget the moment when, minutes before the start of Ironman® Santa Rosa in 2019, I realized that I couldn't wait for the 10 hours of strain and pain that lay ahead and that I was as calm as I would have been before an easy 6-mile run on a random Tuesday. This state of mind could not have been more different from my state of mind before my first Ironman in 2002, when my last words (spoken to my brother Sean in response to the question, "How are you feeling?") before walking to the start line were, "I'm shitting my pants." And the new mind state was not only more pleasant to experience but also more effective, as the older but tougher version of me completed the Ironman distance 25 minutes faster than the younger but weaker version of me.

The keys to my transformation were *meaning* and *practice*. Becoming mentally tough was personally meaningful to me, so I worked hard at it. Friedrich Nietzsche was right: "He who has a why to live for can bear almost any how." But meaning alone didn't suffice to get the job done. I needed to practice being tough, again and again, for many years, gaining a bit of ground each time, like an actor overcoming stage fright not through hypnosis or some other instantaneous cure but by getting back on stage night after night.

According to science, mental toughness is 50 percent genetic, which means it is also 50 percent nongenetic, and for those of us who weren't born tough, it is the desire to be tough that makes us tough. As the 18th-century English poet Horace Smith put it, "Courage is the fear of being thought a coward." Again, Steve Prefontaine's frequent use of the word *guts* comes to mind. In one famous instance, Prefontaine said, "A lot of people run a race to see who is the fastest. I run to see who has the most guts." Regardless of how many or how few toughness genes you were blessed with, only by consciously prizing toughness—perhaps even making it the very point of your racing at certain times—will you fully realize your potential for toughness.

Again, though, it takes practice. One of the most consistent research findings in this area is that, for all of us, mental toughness requires repeated exposure to challenging and stressful situations that test our toughness. It was on the basis of this finding that exercise scientist Lee Crust and psychologist Peter Clough wrote in a 2011 article appearing in the *Journal of Sport Psychology in Action* that "to develop mental toughness, young athletes must be gradually exposed to, rather than shielded from, demanding situations in training and competition in order to learn how to cope." I would only add that the same holds true for adult athletes.

Other experts in the field of mental toughness have developed systematic methods for cultivating this trait in athletes. The two methods that I found especially helpful in building my own mental fitness and have applied successfully with athletes I coach are accountability cues and limit testers.

Accountability Cues

I've long been fascinated by codes, oaths, pledges, credos, and mantras. All of these related tools are used, or can be used, to hold oneself accountable to a certain standard of behavior. Through them, athletes and others transform vague intentions into explicit rules, and therein lies their power. In stressful situations, like when you're struggling in a race and beginning to doubt your ability to achieve your goal, it can be difficult to spontaneously come up with a thought or a snippet of self-talk that delivers just the right message to enable you to hang in there. Different from positive self-talk, accountability cues are more corrective in nature, and they obviate the problem of coming up with a way to stay on track by allowing you to fall back on prepared words that represent the athlete you want to be when the going gets tough.

It's no accident that many elite runners and other top athletes who are celebrated for their toughness have relied on accountability cues. For former marathon world record holder Paula Radcliffe, it was "No limits." For 2:20 marathoner Sara Hall, it's "The well is deep." And for legendary professional cyclist Jens Voigt, it was "Shut up, legs!" Such phrases counteract the panic reflex that threatens to control our thoughts and actions in difficult moments by providing an alternative reflex, not unlike how the mnemonic "Stop, drop, and roll" has saved the lives of many a person whose clothing's caught on fire.

The options are endless: "Never give up." "No excuses." "Be brave." The more personal your chosen accountability cues are—the more they come from the heart, in other words—the more effective they will be in holding you to the standard you've set for yourself. My mantra for my second Ironman was "Don't panic," a choice I made based on the fact that I had hit the panic button more than once in my first Ironman and on the expectation that I would face the same temptation again. Sure enough, I did, but the words I had prepared in advance kept me from repeating the mistake I'd made 17 years before.

With few exceptions, runners who truly, deeply want to be tough use accountability cues in hard workouts and races. All runners engage in some form of self-talk while running, but whereas in the minds of runners who struggle with pacing, self-talk often takes the form of an unstructured shouting match between base instincts and their best self, pacing masters put their best self in charge before the battle even begins through accountability cues.

Limit Testers

Training is more than a vehicle for building fitness. It is also a potential vehicle for building toughness. Each run you do should have a specific fitness-building purpose, but a select few workouts should be set aside for the special purpose of suffering for suffering's sake. I call these workouts limit testers.

A well-designed limit tester subjects the runner to intense suffering but is not so punishing that it does more harm than good physically. This balance can be achieved through workout formats that require you to run as hard as you can for short periods of time. There are two basic ways to run to your limit, both of which were first discussed in Chapter 2: closed loops and open loops. Closed-loop limit testers are runs or run segments with a definite endpoint that are intended to be reached at a maximum effort. Open-loop limit testers are runs that continue to the point of failure.

An example of a closed-loop limit tester is a set of six 1-mile repetitions where the first five are run at a 10K pace and the last mile is completed as fast as possible. Another example is long accelerations, in which runners gradually accelerate from a jog to a full sprint over the course of several minutes. An example of an open-loop limit tester is the Prefontaine, where runners complete alternating 200 m segments at a 1-mile race pace and 1-mile race pace plus 10 seconds per 200 m until they can no longer hold the required paces. All of these limit testers are included in the training plans at the back of this book and also in the library of workouts available at https://www.8020endurance.com.

The ultimate limit tester, of course, is racing itself. Because racing is highly taxing on the body, hence somewhat disruptive to the training process, it must be done sparingly. But shorter races such as 1-mile track events and 5K road events can be done at modest levels of fitness and require less recovery time than longer competitions. It therefore encourages athletes seeking to build toughness or reconnect with their toughness after a prolonged layoff from racing to sprinkle their preparation for important events with short races that serve mainly as limit testers. There's simply no better way to develop a feel for—and push back—one's perceptual limit.

Limit testers in general build toughness in two ways. First, they increase tolerance for the type of discomfort that is experienced in maximal running efforts. This was demonstrated in a 2017 study led by Thomas O'Leary of the UK Ministry of Defense, which found that subjects who completed either 6 weeks of moderate-intensity training or 6 weeks of painful high-intensity training experienced similar improvements in aerobic fitness, but the latter group showed significantly more improvement in an open-loop time-to-exhaustion test and a test of pain tolerance.

The second way in which limit testers increase mental toughness is by enhancing self-efficacy. Runners who routinely make the choice to subject themselves to intense discomfort in workouts come to see themselves differently than those who do not. Specifically, they see themselves as being capable of *choosing* to hurt in pursuit of their running goals. As runners move toward pacing mastery, their running experience seems less and less like something that is happening to them and more and more like something they are making happen. Limit testers are another helpful contributor to this wonderful feeling of sports mastery.

6

Pacing in Training

Mastering pacing is not about learning how to run completely by feel, paying no attention to numbers. It's about finding your limit, which requires a fine calibration of subjective perceptions against objective measurements. Running free does not mean running like a wild horse, by intuition alone. It means knowing what you can do and then doing it. Pacing masters are runners who know how they ought to be feeling 16.6 miles into a marathon, or 12 seconds into their seventh out of ten 60-second hill repetitions, or whatever. In other words, pacing masters aren't just good at reading their perceptions generally; they are good at reading their perceptions as they relate to distance, time, and speed. The best way to develop pacing skill, therefore, is to systematically train this specific ability.

In the preceding chapter, we looked at ways you can develop the key mental traits that underlie pacing skill. Now it's time to shift our focus to the skill itself, discussing ways to improve pacing prowess by calibrating perceptions against measurements. There are three methods that I have found to be especially useful for this purpose: effort-based training, specific repetition, and special pacing challenges.

EFFORT-BASED TRAINING

Effort-based training is just what it sounds like: pacing yourself without the help of a device. It's okay to wear a watch for the purposes of recording data and knowing when to start and finish segments of a structured workout, but in an effort-based run, you're not taking any pacing cues from your watch, relying instead on perceived effort to control your pace. The important thing—whether you choose to leave your device at home or set the display to show only non-pace-related data—is that you give yourself no option to cheat. When runners complain that they're just no good at pacing by feel, it's usually because they've never really tried, and they've never really tried because they can cheat as often as they like by glancing at their wrist. With effort-based training, cheating is not allowed, and it's amazing what a difference it makes for a lot of runners.

"I used to watch my heart rate like a hawk," wrote one such runner on the 80/20 forum after I persuaded him to give the method a try. "It got to where running wasn't fun. So I altogether stopped looking at anything other than time or distance on the easy runs, except for after the fact. Not even worrying about power, pace, or heart rate. Just doing whatever feels easy. It's been liberating not worrying about those things. It feels like the effort is always just right, and running is fun again."

How to Measure Your Effort

In 1982, Swedish psychologist Gunnar Borg wrote a scientific paper in which he claimed that perceived exertion (a.k.a. perceived effort) is "the single best indicator of physical strain." This claim was not well received initially by the exercise scientists whose turf was infringed upon by this claim, but today we know not only that Borg was right but also *why* he was right. As I explained in Chapter 2, it is now established science that perceived effort is the limiting factor in endurance performance. To feel you have reached your limit is to have reached your limit, plain and simple. Not every researcher who clings to the belief that heart rate or oxygen consumption or blood lactate or something else biological is the best indicator of physical strain has died off yet, but they are an endangered species.

Take blood lactate. Suppose you complete a standard, high-intensity, run-to-exhaustion test, at the end of which your blood lactate and perceived effort levels are measured. You then go on a low-carb diet for 2 days and repeat the same test. When you quit this second run to exhaustion, your blood lactate level will be lower than it was the first time. That's because lactate production is affected by carbohydrate availability. But your perceived effort will be unchanged from the first test. Which of these two measures, then, is the more reliable indicator of your limit?

What distinguishes perceived effort from any physiological measure is that it's the only indicator of physical strain that comes straight from its true source, which is the brain. All conscious experiences, including perceived effort, emerge from brain activity. The hardest-working part of the brain during running is the premotor cortex, whose job is to make the body do what the mind wants it to. Brain imaging studies have shown that activity in the premotor cortex tracks closely with perceived effort ratings. This tells us that the primary determinant of how hard exercise feels at a given moment is how hard the brain is working to drive the muscles. Activity in the premotor cortex can be thought of as the brain giving the body a verbal command to move. When that voice is whispering "move," running feels quite easy, and when it's screaming "MOVE!" running feels extremely hard.

If the name Gunnar Borg rings a bell, by the way, it's because you're familiar with the Borg scale of perceived exertion, which went from 6 to 20 originally but has been modified (thankfully) to go from 1 to 10. And if Borg's name doesn't ring a bell, you might remember the three-letter sequence RPE, which stands for rate of perceived exertion and represents the Borg scale's units. Borg created the scale to serve as a way both to test his belief that effort perceptions are the best indicator of physical strain and to monitor and prescribe intensity. This work has continued beyond Borg's own lifetime, and what it has revealed is that runners have no trouble rating their current overall effort on a 1-to-10 scale and that these ratings correlate well with measures of physiological intensity. The consensus today is that, as researchers at Munich Technical University put it in an article appearing in the *European Journal of Applied Physiology*, "Borg's RPE seems to be an affordable, practical and valid tool for monitoring and prescribing exercise intensity, independent of gender, age, exercise modality, physical activity level and [cardiovascular disease] status."

There's only one problem. Scientific studies report average results, which tend to gloss over individual differences. And you'd best believe there are individual differences in perceived effort ratings. I remember reading that when American professional runner and 2:20 marathoner Jordan Hasay was returning to training from an injury, her orthopedist asked her to report her pain level on a 1–10 scale after each run, but he soon abandoned the practice in exasperation when it became clear that Hasay would never rate any pain above a 2. She could be attacked by a swarm of killer bees and still would report level 2 pain, maybe level 1. Similarly, I have observed that not every runner has the same idea of 2 RPE, or 5, or 7, or 10. Some attempt at standardizing the modified Borg scale must be made to ensure that all runners do more or less the same thing when asked to run for 15 minutes at an RPE of 6 or whatever.

The standardized version of the RPE scale that I use with runners was created through a simple process that involved translating the objective, physiological performance targets I normally use to prescribe intensity into perceived effort ratings. A small amount of fudging was required, but that's okay. There's no less fudging involved in intensity targets based on lab testing, which seldom yields the same results twice. So it's no big deal if your RPE marker for a particular physiological threshold is inexact. The only precision that is truly important in running is the ability to find your real limit in competition, and that's exactly what we're aiming for here.

Physiological Anchors

The primary physiological anchor point of my perceived-effort scale (see Table 6.1) is the first ventilatory threshold (VT_1), which is associated with an RPE of 4. This threshold is important because most runners unwittingly do most of their supposed easy running slightly above it, whereas studies have shown that improvements in fitness and performance are greatest when the VT_1 is never exceeded in easy runs and other runs intended to target low intensity. The VT_1 also happens to correspond to the highest intensity at which a runner can close their mouth and breathe through their nose indefinitely. Play around with nose-breathing at different paces until you find the fastest pace you can sustain without the urge to open your mouth and assign an RPE of 4 to it.

The other thresholds are less important with respect to their potential consequences on your fitness development but are nevertheless useful, as they relate to the objective of getting runners on the same page. Your functional lactate threshold (LT) is the highest intensity you could sustain for about 60 minutes in a race. The RPE associated with this intensity is 6. Next comes critical velocity (CV), which is the highest speed at which your body can maintain a relatively

TABLE 6.1 Standardized RPE-based intensity scale

RPE	PHYSIOLOGICAL CORRELATE	TIME LIMIT
1	---	Indefinite
2	---	Indefinite
3	---	Indefinite
4	First ventilatory threshold (VT_1)	5:00:00
5	Steady state	2:00:00
6	Lactate threshold (LT)	1:00:00
7	Critical velocity (CV)	20:00–30:00
8	Maximal aerobic speed (MAS)	6:00
9	---	1:00–5:00
10	Maximal velocity	0:30

stable metabolic state and is sustainable for 20 to 30 minutes, depending on the individual. That might seem like a large range, but in pace terms, we're talking about a few seconds per mile, so minimal fudging is required to associate a one-size-fits-all RPE of 7 with CV. Finally, your maximal aerobic speed (MAS) is the lowest running speed at which your body will max out its capacity to utilize oxygen. In functional terms, this threshold is sustainable for 6 minutes, give or take, regardless of fitness level (though the velocity itself increases with fitness), and it gets an initial RPE of 8.

Everything else is filler. Warm-ups, cooldowns, and active recoveries are tagged with an RPE of 3. This is an effort level you feel you could sustain almost indefinitely on fresh legs. Lower RPEs—specifically 1 and 2—are never targeted in training. Reserve them for walking the dog and climbing the stairs in your home. A 5 RPE correlates roughly with steady-state pace, which is a pace you could sustain for 2 hours or perhaps a bit longer. A 10 RPE is a true maximal effort that cannot be sustained longer than 30 seconds. This leaves RPE 9 to cover everything from a 1-minute max effort to a 5-minute max effort, approximately.

The Fine Print

Effort-based training involves a bit more than strict adherence to this 10-point scale. The first thing you need to understand if you're going to train effectively by perceived effort is that RPE increases over time at *any* fixed intensity. Heck, if you *walk* long enough, your RPE will reach 10 eventually. Hence the RPE assigned to any particular run segment is always an initial rating that serves to set the intensity and is expected to increase as you go, even as the physiological intensity remains constant. In other words, for prescriptive purposes, RPE assumes no prior fatigue. This means that if I ask you to run 12 × 1:00 at RPE 9 with 2:00 active recoveries at RPE 3, your pace for both the intervals and the recoveries should stay the same throughout the workout even though, realistically, by the time you reach the tenth rep, you'd probably have to walk the recoveries to get your RPE down to 3, and when you start the next rep, your RPE will rise above 9 very quickly. It's just a matter of linking each RPE number to a specific pace or intensity that is fixed for the rest of the run.

More generally, there's room for interpretation, contextualization, and common sense in using the 10-point scale. For example, if I asked you to complete an interval set comprising 6 × 2:00 at RPE 8, and on another occasion, I asked you to run 4 × 3:00 at RPE 8, you can and should exploit the fact that this RPE value, like the others in the scale, represents a narrow range, not a point, and run the longer intervals slightly slower than the shorter ones.

Effort-based training does not require you to completely tune out objective performance metrics (i.e., pace and run power). For the most part, you should completely ignore such metrics during RPE-guided runs, but it's okay and even advisable oftentimes to look at your pace and/or power data afterward. This can help you assess your pacing performance and document your progress toward pacing mastery. I'll give you a specific example of how to conduct this sort of post hoc analysis when I discuss long accelerations later in the chapter.

Finally, although it is possible to train effectively for races with RPE-based runs exclusively, I don't believe it's the most effective way to develop pacing skill. There's something to be said for training by pace or power in select workouts where the aim is to exercise precise control over pace. Indeed, such workouts do more than any other to calibrate subjective effort perception to objective reality. And when you feel you've achieved a sufficient level of pacing mastery, you can go back to using pace- or power-based training generally. The only run type that should always be done by perceived effort, in my view, is easy runs. This is because easy runs account for the bulk of any sensible runner's training time, and allowing your pace to fluctuate from day to day based on how you feel is a simple way to fine-tune your training load as you go. Affording yourself this latitude will help you avoid having to make the bigger adjustments to your plan that often result when runners don't listen to their bodies.

SPECIFIC REPETITION

The training style of Japan's elite runners is rather monotonous by the standards of some runners from other places. Pro runners everywhere run a lot, but the Japanese tend to run more than their counterparts in the rest of the world. Australian runner Melissa Duncan wasn't aware of this when she joined the Tokyo-based Shiseido Running Club in 2019, and she got a rude awakening in her first team meeting, where she learned that she and her new teammates would be running three times the next day—and the day after that, and the day after that, up to 200 km (160 miles) per week all told.

In addition to running a lot, Japanese elite runners have a predilection for loop courses. Boston Marathon winner Toshihiko Seko took this approach to an extreme in his 1980s heyday, doing most of his runs—including long runs of up to 40 km—around a 1.3-km loop. That was 40 years ago, but a milder form of the practice remains common today. Japan's top runners tend to cycle through a limited variety of workouts over and over, as the world was reminded when Hitomi Niiya's training log was posted online after she set a national record of 1:06:38 in the 2020 Houston Half Marathon. Those who took the time to scroll through the schedule saw a small handful of workout types, most notably 400-meter and 1000-meter intervals, repeated again and again. A few workouts of other types (hill repetitions, steady-state runs) are mixed in there, but not many.

Japanese-born running coach Nobby Hashizume once explained to me that the emphasis on repetition in the training of his native country's elite runners comes from the predominance of ekidens (team relay road races) in their running culture. Tactical head-to-head racing plays a very small role in these competitions, while steady solo pacing plays a very large role, for which a highly repetitive style of training serves as excellent preparation. It's easy to see why.

When you do certain types of workouts repeatedly, you get to know them intimately, becoming sensitive to ever-finer details of the experience, which enables you to execute the pacing element of the workout with ever-increasing confidence and competence. What's more, this newfound pacing efficacy is to some extent generalizable to the rest of your running. It's sort of like how taking a deep dive into a certain musical artist makes you better at listening to all music.

Additional benefits come from comparing your performance in often-repeated workouts against your performance in races. Over time, these workouts become benchmarks that enable you to set appropriate goals and realistic expectations for races. It doesn't particularly matter which specific workouts you use for this purpose. All that matters is that you do enough of them in the lead-up to a race of a given distance to know how your performance in them correlates to race performance. You're simply doing the workouts, noting your times, racing, and then comparing after the fact, so that the same workouts have predictive value when you do them in the future. In the case of Hitomi Niiya, what she did in bread-and-butter workouts like 400-meter and 1000-meter repeats told her what she could do in her half-marathon, but both the workouts and the race distance could have been different and her use of specific repetition would have had the same effect.

Simplicity is a virtue in such runs. A very basic workout structure facilitates both the process of familiarization and apples-to-apples comparisons between runs of the same type. So much has been written and said about training for running over the decades that those of us who write and speak publicly on the topic feel a certain pressure to create novelty ("Here's an exotic workout you've never seen before!"). An unintended consequence of such novelty bias is that it causes runners to lose sight of the value of straightforward workouts such as 12 × 300 meters at a 3000-meter race effort.

Naturally, the workouts you choose to repeat most regularly need to have some relevance to the race you're training for in terms of their fitness benefits. A 4-hour long run is not the best choice for specific repetition if you're training for a 1500-meter track race, nor is a set of 100-meter sprints the ideal bread-and-butter workout to use in preparing for a 100-mile trail ultramarathon. The specific pace you target in such workouts should at least fall within shouting distance of race pace. You need not—and in fact should not—limit yourself to

How to Run the Perfect Race

just one workout type, though. You'll get that much more out of your use of specific repetition if, like Niiya, you choose at least a couple of workout types, perhaps one targeting an intensity that's faster than race pace for your upcoming event and another targeting an intensity that's about equal to or slightly slower than race pace.

Also, the workouts you use for the purpose of specific repetition should not be identical each time you do them. Instead they should gradually become more challenging so that they keep pushing your fitness level upward. For example, you might start a sequence with 4 × 4:00 at critical velocity, advance to 5 × 4:00 the next time, and add a sixth rep in the third and final workout of the sequence. Note that all of the training plans presented in Chapters 9 through 12 include sequences of bread-and-butter workouts chosen in accordance with the principle of specific repetition.

SPECIAL PACING CHALLENGES

Picture a contest for runners that has the following design: Each contestant stands alone with a "guide" at the start line of a half-marathon. The guide goes first, beginning to make her way through the course at a steady pace that is unspecified, except that the contestant she's partnered with knows it's slower than his own half-marathon race pace. The moment the guide reaches the course's first turn and disappears from sight, the contestant is allowed to start.

His goal is to catch the guide as close to the finish line as possible. Hence the challenge the contestant is faced with is judging the guide's pace in the first 30 or 60 seconds she's visible, considering the distance to be covered, and choosing a pace that's just enough faster than the guide's to close the gap over precisely 13.11 miles. The wrinkle is that the contestant's performance is judged not only by how close to the finish line the catch occurs but also by how even his 1 km split times are throughout the chase, so contestants can't just game the system by closing the distance as quickly as possible and then shadowing the guide until the very end.

It's a wacky format yet straightforward enough to function as a pure test of pacing skill. If 100 different contestants were to complete the challenge on five separate occasions on different courses and with a new guide each time, some would consistently achieve top scores, while others would perform relatively poorly with equal consistency. And you can bet that the top runners would be the same runners who succeeded best in finding their limit in normal races because when you're good at pacing, you're good at pacing. If you're adept at pacing routine workouts and normal races, you're likely to be adept (at least in relation to other runners) at executing novel tests of pacing ability and vice versa.

In the previous section, I made an analogy between developing pacing skill and cultivating an ear for music. My point was that repeated exposure to any particular kind of experience leads to more nuanced perceptions of it, which in turn lead to greater control. But there's just as much to be said for throwing curveballs at perception. In reality, no runner ever truly runs the same race or workout twice. In small ways, at least, each running experience is unique, and for this reason, it takes a certain kind of mental agility to pace well with consistency. Special pacing challenges are designed to improve this aspect of pacing skill.

I must confess that I quite like the half-marathon tracking game I came up with, but it's not terribly practical. Fortunately, there are plenty of other special pacing challenges that can be done anywhere at any time without outside help while also conferring the fitness benefits one seeks in regular workouts. The following are short descriptions of a handful of such formats I've collected and invented over the years, all of which are included in the training plans presented in Chapters 9 through 12. Feel free to create your own special pacing challenges—the options are endless, and the whole idea is to keep challenging your pacing skill with the unfamiliar.

Precision Splitting

These workouts develop your ability to hit the same time—down to the hundredth of a second, if possible—in each interval of a set such as 8 × 400 m or 6 × 800 m. There are two ways to go about it. One is to pick an appropriate target time before the workout and aim to nail it perfectly from start to finish. The other option is to run the first interval by feel, capture your time, and then try to hit the same time in every subsequent rep.

Obviously, this is not a challenge that works for time-based intervals, and I do prefer time-based intervals generally because they are one-size-fits-all. A set of 2-minute intervals at maximal aerobic speed is equally challenging for fast and slow runners alike because both are able to sustain this speed for about 6 minutes straight. But a set of 600 m intervals at MAS is significantly more challenging for slower runners because it takes them longer to cover that distance, so they're coming closer to their limit in each interval. To get a pacing challenge similar to that of precision intervals in a time-based workout, try stretch intervals instead.

Stretch Intervals

This pacing challenge is made up of intervals of a uniform duration in which you aim to cover slightly more distance each time. For example, you might run 10 × 30 seconds uphill, completing the last rep at maximal effort and each preceding rep just a hair slower. The challenge here is to run the first rep at a high effort level that leaves just enough space for nine subsequent increases in speed. To execute this type of workout properly, you will need some way of marking the endpoint of each interval. I like to use brightly colored socks, dropping one at the finish of the first rep, dropping the other at the end of the second rep, retrieving the first on my way back to the starting point for interval number three, and so forth.

Stretch intervals improve pacing skill by challenging you to perceive tiny differences in speed and effort and to regulate your speed and effort with a higher degree of precision than you are accustomed to doing. Most runners find stretch intervals difficult both physically and mentally yet also fun.

Fast-Finish Long Runs

There's a rule I sometimes impose on runners who have a tendency to fade toward the end of long runs. It's called the fastest-mile-last rule, and it works just the way it sounds: The runner is required to complete the last mile (or kilometer) of the run faster than any preceding mile. It's a simple way to encourage runners to be more mindful in their pacing from the outset, making sure they save enough energy to speed up in the homestretch. A majority of the training plans at the back of this book feature time-based long runs with a 5-minute fast finish, but it's the same idea and offers the same benefit.

Mind you, a perfectly executed fast finish is not an all-out effort that leaves you dry heaving at the foot of your driveway but a gentle push resulting in a split time that's a few ticks quicker than the next quickest segment of the run.

Practicing this method habitually will train your mind to think ahead in all of your runs, including races, as pacing masters do.

Long Accelerations

Go out and run for 3 minutes, 6 minutes, or 11 minutes, accelerating continuously the entire time without consulting your watch. This is theoretically doable, as acceleration is something every runner can feel. In fact, accelerating continuously for much shorter periods—say, 10 to 20 seconds—is quite easy. But drawing out a continuous acceleration over several minutes demands a high degree of body attunement and nuanced pace control, and that's what makes long accelerations a terrific special pacing challenge.

In the preceding chapter, long accelerations were presented as a tool for building toughness. And they are that. But they're even more mentally taxing than they are physically challenging, as any runner who's done them can attest. The most common mistake made in executing long accelerations is speeding up too quickly, which results in an "Oh, shit" moment when the runner realizes that, with time still on the clock, they've run out of gears. I call this pacing yourself into a corner. The limit comes more suddenly than most first-timers anticipate. So don't think about accelerating per se. That's too black and white. Think about *accelerating as slowly as possible*—so slowly that it's hard to tell sometimes whether you're truly speeding up or you're making the second-most common error in executing long accelerations, which is plateauing in pace or even slowing down a bit at various points along the way.

Although you are forbidden to monitor your pace when doing a long acceleration, you should record your workout data so you can look at it later and judge your performance. Focus on the pace curve. It should be gently upward sloping from end to end. The likelihood of this happening will be greater if you run your accelerations on a flat route. If you run with a power meter, an undulating route will serve the purpose. In this case, your power curve will give you a better indication than the pace of how you performed.

Relaxed Time Trial

Here's how to do a relaxed time trial: Warm up and then run 5 km or 10 km at a 95 percent effort, aiming to cover the distance 5 percent slower than you would in a race. I started doing relaxed time trials many years ago because they seemed like a good way to sharpen up, build confidence, and dial in my time goal for an upcoming race of the same distance, but I've since come to appreciate relaxed time trials as a special pacing challenge.

The ideal time to do a relaxed time trial is about 2 weeks before a race of the same distance. Your performance is judged by the time delta between the two. If it's exactly 5 percent, you get a lollipop. I've done enough relaxed time trials that I've gotten quite good at them. In my last one, I covered 10 km in 35:08. A couple of weeks later, I ran a 10 km virtual race (this was during the COVID-19 pandemic, so there were no real races to run) in 33:25, which is 4.9 percent faster!

The 5K and 10K distances work best for relaxed time trials because they are long enough to constitute workouts unto themselves but not so long as to leave you worn out and beaten up for 2 or 3 days afterward. I myself have actually done full marathons as relaxed time trials.

Mini Intervals

Few pacing errors annoy me more than that of automatically tuning one's effort to the interval duration regardless of what the workout description calls for. I'll prescribe 5 × 3:00 at 5K race pace, and the runner will simply ignore the pace target and run the intervals as fast as they can without cratering.

"What's the big deal?" you ask. After all, they're still getting a good workout. The big deal is that skillful pacing is all about control, and when athletes are allowed to do everything by reflex, they don't learn control. It's not the non-compliance that bugs me when runners mindlessly tune their effort to interval duration but the mindlessness itself and its consequences.

Mini intervals are a tool I use to break this habit. An example is 60 × 30 seconds on, 30 seconds off, where the "on" segments are run at lactate threshold pace and the "off" segments are run at VT_1 pace. The brevity of the intervals tempts runners to go much faster than the prescribed pace, but if they do, they'll pay dearly (and deservedly!) after 20 repetitions, when they've still got *40* left. Mini intervals all but force runners to make a good-faith effort at compliance, thereby training them in mindful control of pace. After completing them, analyze the data, and judge your performance by the consistency of your pace and how close you got to LT pace in the "on" segments.

DON'T FORGET TO HAVE FUN!

The biggest misstep that I made when I started to teach pacing skill to runners in a programmatic way was unintentionally making some of them feel like every run was a test of some kind. That's no fun, and it had a negative effect on the overall motivation and enjoyment levels of some.

We must never allow our pacing work to spoil the fun of training. As important as it is to be conscious of pace in certain runs that are earmarked for pacing skill development, it's equally important to relegate pacing to the back of your mind in other runs. Pacing skill development is meant to be a project, not an obsession. And the overall process should be rewarding, not frustrating, to which end I urge the runners I work with—and you—to focus on the progress that's being made rather than on how far away pacing mastery seems. You can't run free if your running is in any way a burden.

7

Pacing in Competition

There's a reason I define pacing as the art of finding your limit. More than a few great runners over the years have viewed their races as works of art. Steve Prefontaine (once again) was one such runner, who, while still competing for the University of Oregon, said, "Some people create with words or with music or with a brush and paints. I like to make something beautiful when I run."

It's no accident that the word *performance* is used to refer to what musicians, actors, and other artists do on stage as well as to what runners do in races. For performing artists, there is no amount of rehearsal that guarantees a successful performance before a live audience. It isn't just that they might forget a line or break a string. It's also that, even if everything goes according to script, the performance could be better or worse based on other factors, such as how they're feeling about what they're doing. The greatest performers embrace this uncertainty, relishing the high-stakes nature of performance. They don't want guarantees.

Alas, the same cannot be said of many runners, particularly those who struggle with pacing. Lacking confidence in their ability to solve the unique puzzle that each race presents, these runners would gladly accept an alternate reality in which, if they just did all the necessary work to prepare for a great performance, the performance itself would be automatic. It's a vain wish, however. To find your limit in any given race, you must improvise, working with what you've got that day to feel your way to an outcome that remains undetermined until the moment it happens. Granted, this does mean you have no one but yourself to blame if you blow it. But it also means you get all the credit if you nail it!

Wouldn't you like to create something beautiful when you run? Of course you would. And the only way to do so is to embrace the racing experience as the live solo act that it is. It's like tangoing before a panel of surly judges with a competitive dance partner you've only just met. The many past tangos you've done with other partners will give you a chance to score perfect 10s, but this will only happen if you're able to quickly and effectively read your partner and cooperate with them to create a performance that looks rehearsed. Think of each race you do as a new dance partner, and think of those perfect 10s as your personal performance limit on that day.

A good example of what this looks like in the real world comes from Sarah Crouch, an elite runner with whom I did some training during my summer in Flagstaff with NAZ Elite. The following May, Sarah flew to Grand Rapids to race in the 2018 USATF 25K Championships. Her last several competitive outings had been disappointing, and 4 long years had passed since Sarah set a personal best at any distance. Something had to change, and on the eve of the event, Sarah announced that she would compete "naked," sans watch, which is not unheard of at the professional level (Galen Rupp left his watch at home when he won the 2020 Olympic Trials Marathon) but was unusual for her. Sarah explained her reasoning as follows in a pre-race interview for FloTrack: "I feel that when I'm wearing a watch I'm constantly looking at it. I'm far too much in my own head. So the goal tomorrow is to race just by instinct, and guts."

Intrigued by the experiment, I tuned in to FloTrack's live coverage the next morning. From the moment Sarah first appeared on my computer screen, I knew something special was in the works. She seemed like a different person than the one I had run with less than a year before, running with a striking combination of aggression and serenity, her eyes focused seemingly miles up the road as she dragged eight-time national champion Aliphine Tuliamuk behind her. Incredibly, Sarah passed the half-marathon mark in 1:12:45, just 35 seconds shy of her 4-year-old personal best for that distance, and went on to finish the race in third place. It was a breakthrough performance—Sarah's first podium finish in a national championship race and a huge improvement on her recent racing.

The lesson here is not that runners should never wear watches when they race. In fact, there is no lesson, but through Sarah's story, you can see what's possible when a runner fully accepts the performative nature of racing and allows today's limit to guide her to it. Sarah Crouch wasn't just satisfied with her performance in Grand Rapids; she was ecstatically proud of it, and duly so, because she had created it from nothing.

I want you to be ecstatically proud of your future races, and to that end, I will devote this chapter to sharing my best advice for pacing in competition. The three most common errors in race pacing are (1) bad planning (or not having a plan), (2) not sticking to the plan, and (3) sticking too much to the plan. I'll show you how to avoid each of these errors by applying the principles and methods of optimal pacing I've taught you to each unique race experience to create the best possible performance. We will then wrap up by addressing the important difference between racing for time and racing to beat other runners.

BAD PLANNING OR NO PLAN

Jim Walmsley came into the 2018 Ultra-trail du Mont Blanc (UTMB) in France with big ambitions. Having recently smashed the course record at the Western States 100, Jim wanted to apply the same winning formula at the 106-mile UTMB (where he'd finished fifth in his debut the year before), coming out hot and cooking the competition early. Alas, he cooked himself instead, dropping out at 75 miles.

"I like to think I'm more willing to push into a pace with an unknown outcome," he told *Runner's World* writer Amanda Loudin afterward. "It's both a strength and a weakness, but I feel it sets me up to surprise myself and do things I may not have otherwise thought possible. It can also set me up for a long, hard day with the lowest of lows, too. I love running this way and it's what inspires me to train for these races on the biggest stage."

These words sound like those of a clear-eyed competitor who has no regrets and is not about to change his ways. But after flaming out again at UTMB in 2021 and finishing a disappointing fourth in 2022 after once more setting the pace in the early going, Jim decided that a new approach was needed. The problem, he realized, was his refusal to take the race on its terms, insisting instead on dictating the terms and expecting the formula that worked everywhere else to work at an event that, with its severe terrain and unparalleled level of competition, wasn't like other events. Step one was a full-time relocation to France, where Jim spent countless runs familiarizing himself with the race course. When race day came, he turned his default strategy on its head, going so far as to start the race several rows from the front to keep himself from getting carried away. With "patience" as his mantra, Jim allowed himself to fall 9 minutes behind the leader before clawing his way back, taking the lead for the first time at 59 miles and going on to win in 19:37:43, one of the fastest times in the 21-year history of the event.

The lesson of the story is this: When you start a race, you need to have a plan—and not just a plan but a good one. Jim Walmsley's original plan to win UTMB the same way he won other races was bad because it failed to take due consideration of the event's uniqueness. Only when he developed a new plan that factored in his strengths and weaknesses as well as the realities of the event did he break through and win in his fifth attempt.

I realize that most runners aren't trying to win major ultramarathons, but the same planning rules apply to more modest performance goals like beating your own best time in the annual Independence Day 5K road race. The following five rules will help you avoid experiencing the kind of regret Walmsley did.

Consider Pace First, Time Second

The time goals that runners set for races are often somewhat arbitrary. Round numbers in particular exert a pull that causes many to overreach. So, for example, a runner who thinks they're able to run a 5K in about 21 minutes sets a goal to run 20 minutes, and a runner who feels they're in 3:04 marathon shape sets a goal to break 3 hours. I'm oversimplifying a bit to make a point, but you get the idea.

There's nothing wrong with a 21-minute 5K runner dreaming of running a 20-minute 5K or with a 3:04 marathoner wanting to run a sub-3-hour marathon eventually. The problem is that a runner who's in 21-minute 5K shape today and starts a 5K at a 20-minute pace is likely to finish in 22 minutes, and a runner who's ready to run a 3:04 marathon today and starts out on pace to run 2:59 is likely to finish in 3:14—or not at all. If you want to find your limit in your next race, your goal should be based on a clear-eyed reading of your current ability. This requires that you forget about round numbers—and indeed about finish times in general—for the moment and instead focus on pace. Ask yourself what the fastest pace is that you could sustain for the full distance of your upcoming race, and then use your answer to project a finish time. It's a small difference in orientation, but it's far more likely to yield a goal that represents your present limit.

If you're currently the round-number type of goal setter, chances are you haven't put much thought into the process by which you set goals. A certain number just sort of pops into your head a couple of weeks before the race, and it feels about right, so that's your goal. Pace-based goal-setting, by contrast, is infused throughout the entire training process. Day by day, you ask yourself, "What is this run telling me about the fastest pace I could sustain for the full distance of my upcoming race?" As a result, by the time you settle on a final goal, the number you pick has a solid basis. Benchmark workouts are especially helpful in this regard.

Use Benchmark Workouts to Refine Your Goal

As I mentioned in Chapter 6, any run you do can tell you something about your current fitness, but certain workouts tell you more, especially as they relate to an upcoming race. To fulfill their purpose, such benchmark workouts need to have some relevance to the race they precede, and they must also be familiar enough from prior experience to provide a basis for comparisons. Obviously, it helps if the race distance you're targeting is itself at least somewhat familiar as well.

For example, long runs containing extended efforts at anticipated marathon race pace (e.g., 10 miles easy plus 10 miles at marathon pace) are commonly used as a benchmark workout prior to marathon competition. These workouts are challenging enough that they shouldn't be done very often, but even one big marathon-pace workout done before a marathon will give the runner who does it something to go on when interpreting the results of the next big marathon-pace run performed ahead of a second marathon.

Here are examples of useful benchmark workouts for other popular race distances:

5K: 5 × 1K at estimated 5K race pace / 400 m jog recovery
10K: 6 × 1 mile at estimated 10K race pace / 400 m jog recovery
Half-marathon: 3 × 3 miles (or 5K) at estimated half-marathon pace / 1:00 rest
Marathon: 10 miles easy, 10 miles at estimated marathon pace

Benchmark workouts don't have to be done at your estimated current pace for a particular race distance. The 5K workout above could serve just as well as a benchmark workout for a 10K race if you've done enough of both. Interval workouts targeting maximal aerobic speed have been used with good success as performance benchmarks for 5K races, as have runs focused on critical velocity by runners training for 10Ks and half-marathons. And don't forget about relaxed time trials, as discussed in Chapter 6. The two main criteria for all such runs are relevance and familiarity. Any run becomes familiar with repetition, of course, and relevance is broadly defined in running. Even milers need stamina, and even marathoners need speed.

Aim for Incremental Improvements

In 2007, Haile Gebrselassie set a new world record of 2:04:26 in winning the Berlin Marathon. The first thing he said after crossing the finish line was, "I can run faster." The following year, Geb returned to Berlin and bettered his mark, running 2:03:58—a hair more than 1 second per mile faster than last time.

As this example illustrates, it's easier to know you can go faster than it is to know how fast you can go. In fact, it's infinitely easier, as it is simply impossible for any runner to know how fast they can ultimately go at any race distance. So instead of setting goals based on your best guess as to how fast you can go, just aim for incremental improvement. If, for example, you've run three half-marathons and your best and most recent time was 1:44:14, use this number as a baseline for setting your next goal. If your current training suggests you're ready to make a small step forward, then shoot to lower your mark by 1 to 2 seconds per mile. If you've experienced a breakthrough in fitness since your last half, set the bar a little higher.

You don't always have to be fitter to seek incremental improvements. Haile Gebrselassie wasn't any fitter when he set his second marathon world record at age 36 than he was when he set his first one the year before. He just had the advantage of having already run a marathon in 2:04:26, which gave him a solid basis for believing he could squeeze a few more seconds out of himself. The beauty of incremental improvement is that repetition works magic, enabling runners to go faster even after they've stopped getting "better," coaxing them through the last few purely mental steps toward their ultimate limit.

The weakness of the incremental-improvement approach is that it demands patience, and it assumes you'll have many bites at the same apple—whether it's half-marathons or anything else. But what if your next race is at a distance you've never done, or you specialize in 100-milers, where you only get so many bites at the apple? In these cases, the incremental-improvements approach won't be as useful. Simple as that.

Consider the Course and Conditions

Jim Walmsley is hardly alone in having failed to properly account for course conditions in setting and pursuing a race time goal. Too many runners set goals that assume an easy course and favorable conditions and then apply that goal to an event that has a less-than-easy course and is likely to take place in less-than-perfect conditions. There's nothing wrong with using a "perfect world" scenario as your starting point in the goal-setting process, but this number should be treated as just that: a starting point that is subject to future modification based on specific discrepancies (topography, terrain, winds, temperature and humidity, and elevation, in particular) between a perfect world and the one you'll be racing in.

When cyclist Bradley Wiggins broke the world record for the 1-hour time trial at a London velodrome in 2015, he adjusted his goal from 16.1 seconds per lap to 16.4 seconds per lap at the last moment based on an unexpectedly high barometric pressure reading. A solo cycling time trial performed in a velodrome is a sufficiently controlled experiment that such precision is possible, whereas in most running events, there's a little more guesswork involved. Tools such as the Run S.M.A.R.T. Project's running calculator and Stryd's race prediction feature can help you quantify the anticipated effect of weather and elevation gain on your race pace. Accounting mathematically for other factors, such as strong winds and muddy trails, is more difficult. The runners who do the best job of adjusting their pace to unfavorable conditions of all kinds seldom bother with calculators. Instead they simply start their races with a general expectation of running slower than normal and then *feel* their way to the appropriate pace as they go.

"How is this done?" you ask. It's done the same way good pacing is always done. Runners who succeed in finding their limit despite unfavorable conditions take the race on its own terms, asking themselves throughout it, "Can I sustain this effort the rest of the way?" All runners do this to an extent, but pacing masters do it in a more focused way, actively listening to their perception of effort rather than passively hearing it, as less skilled pacers do. By actively studying their subjective effort, pacing masters not only are better able to answer the all-important sustainability question assuredly but also are able to draw deeper learning from each race, so their answers are even more assured in the next one. A less skilled pacer cannot instantly become a pacing master by emulating their practice of really tuning in to their effort during races, but they can begin to close the gap in this fashion.

By the way, the correct answer to the question "Can I sustain this effort the rest of the way?" (as former 1-hour cycling time trial world record holder Chris Boardman has noted) is not "Yes" but "Maybe." Surprised? Think about it: If you answer "Yes" to this question, meaning you're *sure* the effort is sustainable, then you're all but sure to fall short of your real limit. Keep in mind that to succeed in finding your limit in a race is to just barely escape hitting the wall before you finish, and there's just no way to flirt so closely with disaster without running in a state of uncertainty most of the way. The risk of actually hitting the wall with this approach is minimal because the moment the runner's "Maybe" tilts too far in the direction of "No," warning of impending disaster, they slow down immediately, before it's too late. In regulating their effort during races, pacing masters deliberately seek the narrow zone of uncertainty that lies between knowing they can keep up their current pace and knowing they can't. This chosen uncertainty is very different from the cluelessness of the novice runner, who has no earthly idea whether they're running too fast or too slow or just right. It's a definite "Maybe," if you will. While the runner does not know for sure if they can sustain the effort, they do know that if they're running too fast or too slow, it's not by much.

When a race you're doing is similar in most respects to others of its kind that you've done in the past, you can pace your way through it by regulating your effort based on your knowledge of how you should be feeling at each point along the way. Suppose there's a half-marathon you've run twice before, but in your third go at it, you're forced to complete it under a heavy downpour. In this case, you'll want to make sure your core effort level is the same at 4 miles, at 7 miles, and so forth as it was in prior dry years (assuming you paced those races well), letting the actual numbers take care of themselves rather than keying them off based on some prior calculation.

Such comparative adjustments are less useful in races that are so unique in design that they really can't be compared to other races of the same distance. Kilian Jornet's course record at the Hardrock 100 (22:41:35) is more than 7 hours slower than Jim Walmsley's course record at the Western States 100, not because Jornet is an inferior runner or Hardrock a less competitive race but because the course is far more difficult. A runner who is competing in either of these events for the first time will need to draw on their experience in a general way when answering the question, "Is this effort sustainable?" When planning for extreme races of this sort, you can set rough expectations for your performance by studying historical results. How have runners of similar ability fared in this particular event in past years? Obtaining this information will make you slightly less reliant on perceptions in the early part of the race.

Don't Be Afraid to Make a Mistake

Having a bad race due to poor pacing is not the end of the world—unless it's the Worlds End Ultramarathon in Pennsylvania's Loyalsock State Forest, in which case it's the end of the world even if your pacing is nearly perfect. Always remember that pacing mistakes are grist for the mill of pacing skill development. Yes, it's disappointing—and sometimes downright painful—to hit the wall in a race as a result of misjudging your limit. But each of these experiences has the potential to teach you a lesson that will help you pace better next time.

I say "has the potential" because learning from pacing errors is not automatic. As the philosopher John Dewey wrote, "We do not learn from experience. . . . We learn from reflecting on experience." To avoid repeating the same pacing mistake over and over, you need to reflect on what you did wrong and then take a conscious intention to do otherwise into your next race. This is where decision tracking comes in. After each race, evaluate your pacing decisions with a critical eye, flag the mistakes, and ask yourself what you could have done differently to produce a better overall performance. You can't go back in time, but you can ensure that history doesn't repeat itself.

NOT STICKING TO THE PLAN

Professional triathlete Jesse Thomas came into the 2016 Ironman World Championship with a solid plan. On the basis of prior experience at the Ironman distance as well as recent training performance, he had identified a power target that he intended to sustain throughout the bike leg. A strong runner (he'd won state championships in track and cross country in high school and earned all-American status in the same sports at Stanford University), Thomas needed to ride hard enough to avoid giving up too much ground to the competition but not so hard that his legs had nothing left for the marathon, and his power target struck this balance.

As I say, it was a sound plan. But when he got out onto the bike course and found himself being left behind by übercyclists Sebastian Kienle and Michael Weiss, Thomas cast aside his pre-race strategy and gave chase. Upon reaching the 60-mile mark in the hilltop village of Hawi, Thomas discovered that his average power output up to that point exceeded not just the target he'd set but also his average power in a recent race of half the distance, Ironman 70.3 Santa Cruz.

"And then I just completely crumbled," Thomas told a reporter for *Triathlete* after his disappointing 16th-place finish. "It was a long, long, long day."

Sound familiar? Long days are as common in running as they are in triathlon. All too often, runners arrive at the start line with a well-thought-out pacing plan for the race, only to crumple it up and go faster than intended, whether in reaction to the athletes around them, or as a panic response to an early setback such as having a shoelace come untied, or even just because they feel unexpectedly terrific. Assuming the plan was indeed the right one, such spontaneous departures from script seldom end well, as Jesse Thomas can attest. It's almost as if the you who plans for the race is different from the you who does the race, a less rational version of yourself addled by adrenaline, stress, and competitive juices.

To avoid letting the you who races abandon the plan created by the you who prepares, take a cue from brave Ulysses, that hero of ancient Greek literature. In Homer's *Odyssey*, Ulysses resists falling prey to the Sirens' song by having himself tied to the mast of his boat. That is essentially what you need to do to yourself in committing to your pacing plan for the next race. Take a mental step back from the plan itself and vow to stick to it unless something happens during the race that truly requires you to make an adjustment. This note to your future self will bind you to the mast of your plan when you're tempted to stray from it.

A historical counterpoint to Jesse Thomas's "long, long, long day" at the 2016 Ironman World Championship was Mark Allen's performance at the same event

19 years earlier. It was Allen's swan song as a professional triathlete, a do-or-die attempt to match his former rival Dave Scott's record of six world titles at age 37. Allen's plan for the bike leg was to keep his heart rate at or below 150 beats per minute, a number that, like Thomas's power target, he'd arrived at through experience. In the early miles, Allen lost his lead to a pair of younger Germans, the strongest of whom, Thomas "Hell on Wheels" Hellriegel, eventually built a seemingly insurmountable advantage of 13:31 over the five-time champion. But the reason Allen fell so far behind wasn't that he couldn't go faster. Rather, he lost ground because he chose not to go faster, knowing that sticking to his plan gave him the best chance of winning, regardless of what anyone else did. Resisting the temptation to push harder wasn't easy, but Allen's Ulysses-like discipline was rewarded when a grimacing Hellriegel cracked during the marathon and Allen slid past him and into history.

Remember Mark Allen the next time you're tempted to crumple up your pacing plan midrace.

STICKING TOO MUCH TO THE PLAN

I'll stop picking on Jesse Thomas in a minute, but before I do, I'd like to share something that was said by the winner of the 2016 Ironman World Championship, Jan Frodeno, who finished more than 26 minutes ahead of Thomas on that "long, long, long day." "On race day," Frodeno told Slowtwitch reporter Timothy Carlson, "statistics and numbers all really go to shit." In other words, you can plan all you want, but you'd better be ready to scrap it if the reality you confront in the race is different from the one your plan assumed.

At first blush, Frodeno's sentiment might seem to contradict the advice I just gave you to stick to your pacing plan in races, as Mark Allen did so successfully in 1997. But remember the qualifier: "unless something happens during the race that truly requires you to make an adjustment." It was this caveat that Frodeno was referring to in his colorful post-race remark. To find your limit in a race, you must first have a good plan, and then you must have the discipline to resist emotionally driven temptations to abandon the plan, but you must also be willing to depart from your target numbers if circumstances create a need to do so. And as Jan Frodeno would tell you, in most races, it becomes necessary at some point to improvise, at least in small ways.

I'll give you a personal example of the consequences of sticking to a plan too stubbornly and the rewards of improvising intelligently midrace. In 2002, I ran the Long Beach Marathon in the hope of finishing in 2:45, or 1 minute faster than my personal best. I started at the required pace of 6:18 per mile and held it consistently as I made my way through the pancake-flat course, but around mile 8, the pace began to feel harder than it should have, and my gut told me to slow down. But a second instinct overruled my gut, and I stuck to the plan, with the result that I hit the wall at 21 miles and walked the last 3 miles, finishing in 3:11:16.

Seven years later, I ran the Silicon Valley Marathon with the goal of finishing in 2:39, having recently recorded a half-marathon time that made this goal very reasonable. I started the race at the required pace of 6:05 per mile and held it consistently, but around mile 6, the pace began to feel harder than it should have, and my gut told me to slow down. Right on cue, a second instinct urged me to press on. This time, however, I heeded my gut and eased back to a pace that felt more realistic. The result was that, at 21 miles, I had enough energy left to speed up again, and I finished in 2:41:29, missing my goal but still achieving a new personal best.

Remember that the purpose of a pacing plan is not to carry it out no matter what but to help you achieve a successful race and be open to the possibility that achieving a successful race will require you to modify or even abandon your plan on the fly. These decisions aren't always easy. Sometimes it's hard to know which voice to trust among those squabbling inside your head. I doubt I would have made the good decision I did in the Silicon Valley Marathon if I hadn't made bad decisions like the one I made in the Long Beach Marathon 7 years earlier. Your chances of making the right decision in these difficult moments will be greater if you understand exactly what's happening in them, as you now do.

RACING FOR POSITION

If you want a better understanding of the difference between racing for time, which has been our topic up to this point, and racing for position, which entails trying to finish ahead of other runners, watch the 2016 Olympics men's 1500 m final. The metric mile, as it is known, goes all the way back to the first modern Olympics in 1896 and is almost always a tactical affair, which is a diplomatic way of saying slow. That's because the person who is leading after the first or second of the race's 3.75 total laps seldom wins, so nobody wants to lead, and the pace suffers accordingly. But this particular race was an extreme case.

American Matthew Centrowitz came to Rio as the reigning indoor world champion and a strong medal contender. As such, he did not want to bear the burden of leading any more than the other finalists, but that's precisely where he found himself after the usual sprint for position over the first 100 meters. Centro's medal aspirations were far from dashed at this point, but they soon would be if he either ran too hard and used up all his energy while allowing the other runners to cruise in his slipstream or ran too slow and allowed himself to get boxed in by competitors passing him on the outside. The solution he arrived at was to run slow enough (66 seconds for lap one, 69 seconds for lap two) to tempt other racers to pass him and then abruptly speed up each time a runner tried to do so.

The result was one of the most tactically brilliant running performances I have ever witnessed. Knowing that his competitors were only willing to gamble so much on a bid to seize the lead before the last lap, Centro accelerated as much as necessary to cause each succeeding aspirant to think better of it and fall back. His own gamble was to exert the least effort possible to retain the lead no matter what, even going so far as to throw a couple of elbows at indoor 1000 m world record holder Ayanleh Souleiman as he tried to overtake the American in lap three.

Predictably, all hell broke loose when the bell rang, signaling the final lap. Now everyone was willing to risk everything to pass Centrowitz, who was no less motivated to fight them off, and though Souleiman was able to briefly nose ahead of him on the outside, he couldn't close the deal by moving to the rail, and within seconds, Centro was back ahead, where he remained all the way to the finish. His winning formula was utterly original—leading from the very first step until he stopped the clock at 3:50.00, a time that would be surpassed 3 weeks later by the top four finishers in the final of the Paralympic men's 1500 m T13.

The three keys to racing successfully for position—all exemplified by Matthew Centrowitz's Rio performance—are (1) playing to your strengths, (2) using the runners you're trying to beat to your own best advantage, and (3) running *your* race.

Play to Your Strengths

Each runner has a different combination of strengths and weaknesses than other runners of similar overall ability. Hence if you want to finish ahead of them in a race, you must try to neutralize their strengths with yours. I used to coach a trail runner who had a preternatural gift for bombing down technical descents at high speeds without face-planting. Recognizing this strength, we strategized in a way that enabled him to win races by dropping competitors on early descents and using later descents to overtake competitors he'd allowed to get away from him on preceding climbs and flatter sections. Consider your relative strengths as a runner and how to exploit them in individual races against particular competitors you'll face at those events.

Use Other Runners

In everyday life, it is considered unscrupulous to use other people. In competitive running, however, you're a sucker if you don't! Think of the runners you're trying to beat as objects that you can manipulate in certain ways to increase your chances of finishing ahead of them. An extreme example of this mentality comes from my friend and fellow running coach James McKirdy, who was one of Connecticut's top decathletes in his high school days. In his senior outdoor track season, McKirdy came into the final event of the state championship—the 1500-meter run—in third place, 113 points behind leader Josh Fournier and needing to beat him soundly to claim the title. Prior to the race, McKirdy's coach told him to forget everything he knew about smart pacing and run the first lap ridiculously fast, knowing that Fournier, who was more of a sprint specialist, would mark him closely and pay the price later. More than willing to give this unconventional strategy a try, McKirdy completed the opening 400-meter circuit in 61 seconds (or 5 seconds faster than Matthew Centrowitz in the 2016 Olympics), with Fournier glued to his heels. Sure enough, as McKirdy lost steam, Fournier imploded, eventually staggering across the finish line 33 seconds behind the wily winner.

As a coach today, James McKirdy defines *racing* (meaning racing for position) as affecting how someone else performs with your decisions. This is exactly what I mean by using other runners to your own best advantage. The example I just provided is over the top, but there are lots of other specific decision types that you can use to affect the performance of other runners in competition. These include surging to test the legs of a competitor you're currently matching strides with, tucking in behind other runners to let them do the extra work of blocking the wind and setting the pace, masking your discomfort behind a poker face to sow doubt in the mind of a competitor, and exaggerating your discomfort (i.e., playing possum) to make another runner overconfident before you strike.

Run Your Race

The flip side of controlling other runners in such ways is not allowing them to control you. Running your own race means pacing your race in a way that best serves your competitive interests regardless of what your competitors do. I witnessed a good example of this strategy at the 2007 USATF Cross Country Championships in Boulder, Colorado. Dathan Ritzenhein took the men's senior race out hard, breaking away from the lead pack just 1 km into the 12K race. Alan Culpepper, judging the pace too aggressive, elected to let him go, a decision that resulted in Ritzenhein gapping him by 20 seconds over the next 3 km. But in lap four of six, Ritz began to falter, and Culpepper's self-control was rewarded with a dominating 26-second victory.

In the heat of battle, it can be difficult to make the correct split-second decision in reaction (or nonreaction) to something another runner does. In some instances, it's in your best interest to cover a competitor's surge; in others, it's best to let the runner go. You won't always make the right decision, but if you run each race with the intent to control your performance regardless of others' actions, and if you use post-race decision tracking to assess your tactical decisions, you will eventually get to a place where you (almost always) do the right thing.

8

Macropacing

Catching COVID-19 wasn't the only thing I did in Atlanta in February 2020. I also watched the US Olympic Team Trials women's and men's marathons, which took place the day before my last official race. It's hard to think of a better way to get psyched up for competition. Tens of thousands of running fans crowded the sidewalks to witness big names like Galen Rupp and Des Linden as well as up-and-comers including Jake Riley and Molly Seidel take their best shot at qualifying for the Tokyo Olympics. It was a thrilling experience, and among the biggest thrills for me, as a 48-year-old, still-competitive runner, was seeing 43-year-old Abdi Abdirahman qualify for his fifth Olympics with a third-place finish in the men's race.

I had followed Abdi's career from the beginning, and I had even run with him a few years earlier, so I wasn't quite as surprised as some people were by his performance in Atlanta. I knew the answer to the question many folks were asking about Abdi after the race: "What's his secret?"

In a word, pacing.

Until this point I've been writing as if pacing happens only within individual runs, but that's only one kind of pacing, which we can now classify as *micropacing*. If micropacing is the "goal-directed distribution and management of effort across the duration of an exercise bout," *macropacing* is the goal-directed distribution of effort across a full training cycle or even an entire competitive running career. Within a single run, pacing enables a runner to find their present limit.

Over longer time spans, a slightly different application of the same basic aptitude allows runners like Abdi Abdirahman to reach and sustain their *ultimate* limit.

Macropacing is not simply an extended version of race pacing, however. Side-by-side graphs of optimal race pacing and optimal career pacing would look rather different. In race pacing, as we know, the watchword is *steadiness*. A graph of a well-paced race takes the shape of a horizontal line with gentle undulations and perhaps a spike at the very end marking the finishing kick. A graph of Abdi Abdirahman's entire running career, by contrast, would look more like an upward-sloping sine wave, with sharp dips indicating the 3- to 4-week breaks he took after each training cycle, occasional peaks representing periods when he was doing as much work as his body could absorb (like when I met him a few weeks before the 2017 New York City Marathon), and longer, flattish segments between these peaks and valleys representing an overall pattern of consistency (week after week, month after month, and year after year of speed sessions every Tuesday or Wednesday, tempo runs every Friday, and long runs every Sunday). In short, effective macropacing is a matter of being steady *but not too steady*. If condensed into a single run, the career of Abdirahman and every other runner who just keeps rolling along, season after season, would take the form of a brisk jog broken up by brief accelerations to full speed and occasional dead stops.

You don't have to be Abdi Abdirahman to make five Olympic teams. Wait a minute—yes, you do! That's not what I meant to say. What I meant to say is that most of the macropacing errors runners make can be avoided by following the example of runners like Abdi. If you were to receive advice on macropacing directly from such a runner, they would tell you six things:

1. Be patient.
2. Don't get greedy.
3. Be balanced.
4. Do it your way.
5. Don't let yourself go.
6. Stay in love.

My advice is the same, though I might need more words to express it.

BE PATIENT

Sara Hall ran her first marathon in Los Angeles in 2015, 1 month before her 33rd birthday. Hall was then well along in a successful professional running career that included appearances at the Pan Am Games, the World Indoor Championships, and the World Cross Country Championships. But the marathon is a different animal. Struck by leg cramps in the middle miles, she hobbled across the finish line in 2:48:02.

Eight months later, in Chicago, Hall improved her marathon time to 2:31:14. The following year, she took another minute off her personal best. In 2017, she lowered her PB twice more, going from 2:28:26 in Tokyo to 2:27:21 in Frankfurt. Hall's lone marathon in 2018, held in out-of-the-way Ottawa, was yet another incremental improvement: 2:26:19. In Berlin the next fall, she dropped her time to 2:22:16, and in 2020, at age 37, Hall won the Marathon Project in 2:20:32, the second-fastest time ever run by an American woman.

After setting the last of these marks, Hall told *New York Times* writer Lindsay Crouse, "We can be an instant-gratification culture, but I've had to cultivate a long-term approach to my career. I figured as long as I could keep working on my craft, chipping away, finding joy in the mundane, then that had to be enough." This patient mindset is a requirement for successful macropacing. Progress can't be rushed in running. Improvement often does come quickly in the beginning, but years of methodical "chipping away" (a phrase that was also used by macropacing master Ben Bruce in reference to his own progression) are required to fulfill the last percentage of a runner's potential.

Running tends to attract patient people and cultivate patience in the people it attracts. It's not patience most runners lack but rather an understanding of how to exercise their patience to achieve long-term improvement. Sara Hall lowered her marathon time by 28 minutes over a span of 5 years. Stated like that, it seems like a big leap, but Hall didn't make any leaps in the process of fulfilling her marathon potential. She did not attempt to radically increase her training load or rethink her whole approach to training in search of enormous improvements. Instead, she learned from each marathon cycle, applied what she learned to the next one, and raised the bar a little higher. This is the right formula for manifesting patience in the career arc of any runner.

DON'T GET GREEDY

Drew Hunter returned home to Boulder, Colorado, from Oslo, Norway, in June 2019 with a shiny new PB of 7:39 for 3000 meters and plenty of time to rest a sore right foot he'd acquired while in Europe before he needed to sharpen up for the USATF Outdoor Championships in late July. But the 21-year-old was so hyped up about his soaring fitness that instead of resting, he dove straight back into heavy training, with predictable results. Within a few weeks, Hunter's foot pain had intensified to the point where he was forced to reduce his run frequency to three times per week. Remarkably, he was still able to qualify for the World Athletics Championships in the 5000-meter event, but when he went out to celebrate the achievement with his teammates, he couldn't even put weight on the foot, and he was later forced to withdraw from the competition.

"The biggest thing I've learned this year is to not get too greedy with mileage," Hunter told *Runner's World* writer Hailey Middlebrook in the wake of this disappointment. "Runners have this mindset that more is always better, and that if I'm doing well on 'X' mileage, that I'll be even faster if I do more. But that's not the case."

The British term *purple patch* refers to a period when everything is going right for an athlete. They're nailing every workout, feeling fit, and enjoying the process. It is extremely tempting at these times to keep pushing for more, but doing so almost always leads to regret. Purple patches never last long. They can't because they occur when a runner is very close to peak fitness, which is not a sustainable state. Too often, runners become intoxicated by how well they are running and make a bad decision, either training harder to see if they can get even fitter or ignoring signs that their bodies are at their limits (as Drew Hunter did).

When a purple patch is well timed, a runner is able to complete their peak race in good health and with supreme fitness. But some then get greedy and try to extend their purple patch, teeing up another race to run when they should follow Abdi Abdirahman's example and take a break. These efforts to milk a fitness peak rarely turn out well.

It is only human to get excited when you're killing it in training. But a part of you should also be wary when you enter a purple patch. Know that it can't last long. Enjoy the experience, and don't risk spoiling it—or worse, delaying your next opportunity to hit a purple patch—by trying to go for more.

BE BALANCED

There is a common misconception that the greatest athletes are completely obsessed with their sport and make little room in their lives for anything else. Although some such athletes do exist, most of the top runners I've gotten to know are strikingly balanced. A good example is Kellyn Taylor, another member of the NAZ Elite team with whom I trained in 2017. Taylor is also a good example of a macropacing master, having set her personal-best times for 5000 meters, 10,000 meters, the half-marathon, and the marathon between the ages of 31 and 34 after achieving no small measure of success earlier in her career.

The furthest thing from a running geek, or the type of runner who consumes lots of running media and spends a lot of time talking about running, Kellyn puts the sport completely out of her mind when she's not actively engaged in it. Her top priority is parenting her daughter, Kylyn, who was born when Kellyn was just getting started in her professional running career, as well as a number of foster children that she and her husband, Kyle, have taken into their home over the years. During the time I spent with Taylor and her teammates in Flagstaff, she was deeply immersed in training to become a professional firefighter, a commitment that absorbed tremendous amounts of time and energy. Understandably, Taylor was usually the last runner to arrive for a team workout and the first one to leave after completing it.

You might think this busy, multidimensional lifestyle would be a recipe for poor running, but Taylor's results speak for themselves. And although I can't think of another elite runner who is also a firefighter and a foster parent, balanced human beings are the norm at the highest level of all sports, not just running. Evidence of this comes from an analysis conducted by the Australian Institute of Sport's Personal Excellence program, which focuses on the holistic development of athletes with the goal of maximizing their overall well-being. Program director Megan Fritsch gathered information on the makeup and performance of the Australian Olympic Team in the 2008 and 2012 Summer Games. Interestingly, she found that in both Beijing and London, student athletes were more likely than other athletes to win medals, with student athletes accounting for 40 percent of the 2012 Australian Olympic team and 63 percent of the medals brought home from London. Of course, student athlete status is not a guarantee of life-sport balance, but it is a serviceable stand-in for the purposes of this type of analysis.

The idea that caring a little less about running and a little more about other parts of life yields better long-term running performance is somewhat counter-intuitive. How does it work? Psychologists who've looked at this question have identified a few different reasons. One is simply that balanced athletes are happier, and happier people perform better in any activity they're passionate about. Athletes are human beings, after all, not exercise machines, and human beings have many facets. An athlete can pretend they have only one facet by focusing exclusively on one of them—sport—but the fact of the matter is that they do have other facets, which then whither from neglect, weakening the foundation of overall well-being that athletic performance depends on.

In an interview conducted for the Marathon Handbook after he won the 1974 Commonwealth Games Marathon, English runner Ian Thompson said, "I was happy about a lot of other things in life besides my running. Everything was clicking, and I was in a relaxed frame of mind—which is ideal." These words hold true for every runner. If you want to run your very best, you must fit running into your life in a way that makes you happy with a lot of other things besides your running. In fact, the mere temptation to allow running to completely dominate a person's life is a pretty good indication that the person isn't happy in the first place. Submitting to this temptation will only make things worse. I've been known to tell my athletes that if all they care about is running, their best move is to start caring about other things because doing so will aid their running.

Becoming unbalanced in the direction of sport also tends to negatively impact self-esteem and confidence, which in turn harms performance. A bad race is less likely to strike a blow to a runner's self-esteem and confidence if that race comes the day after the runner aced a chemistry exam or was named Employee of the Week or saw their son give his first piano recital. As these examples show, runners with balanced lives have more sources of positive self-esteem and confidence than runners whose identity is completely enmeshed in the sport. In much the same way that a diverse stock portfolio reduces the risk of being dragged down financially by one bad investment, having a balanced life reduces the risk of being dragged down emotionally by disappointment or failure in one area.

Balanced runners are also at a lower risk of overdoing their training. It's easy to see why. Suppose you quit your job for the sake of turning pro and focusing exclusively on running. The first week is likely to be dominated by feelings of excitement, freedom, and hope. But by Thursday of week 2, you might find yourself sitting on the sofa at three o'clock in the afternoon, bored, having already run twice, lifted weights, and stretched, and think, *I suppose it couldn't hurt to kill some time with a little light crosstraining . . .*

This is why actual professional runners like Kellyn Taylor maintain balanced lives despite having the freedom to go all-in with running. Taylor doesn't have time to overtrain. Heck, she doesn't even have time (or at least doesn't feel she has time) for the fancy mobility exercises that her teammates and other elite runners do before every run. She just shows up and goes, which might not be the best thing from a purely physiological perspective, but again, her results speak for themselves.

Beyond making it harder to overtrain, having a rich life outside of running increases training efficiency. When you have only so much time and energy to devote to your training, you are motivated to make the most of every minute. It's a version of Parkinson's Law—the idea that one's work expands to fill the time available to get it done. Aware that the obverse is true too, savvy corporations use project deadlines and time restrictions as a means to force employees to tighten up their practices in ways that increase the overall quality of their work. You can do the same with your training by strictly compartmentalizing running in the context of your life. As the saying goes, "If you want to get something done, ask a busy person."

DO IT YOUR WAY

The people of Maine are known for their stubborn independence. In this respect, Joan Benoit Samuelson is a "Down-Easter" through and through. Her high school didn't have a girls varsity cross country or track team, so she ran with the boys. When she turned pro, Nike tried to convince her to move to Oregon, where she could train with other high-caliber athletes, but she refused, choosing instead to run alone in her beloved home state. She had a coach (the highly regarded Bob Sevene), but she didn't take much direction from him, preferring to "train by the seat of her pants," as she put it to me in a 2010 interview.

Joan is best known, of course, for winning the 1984 Olympic Women's Marathon. Only 27 years old at the time, she was expected to defend her title 4 years later in Seoul, but she turned down the opportunity in favor of raising a family. Having made this choice, Joan was expected to retire from elite running, but she chose instead to make a number of sporadic comebacks, finishing ninth in the 2000 Olympic Trials Marathon at 43, qualifying for the Olympic Trials Marathon again at 50, and setting an age-group national marathon record of 2:49:09 at 52. Still going strong in her late sixties, Joan won her age group at the 2022 London Marathon.

There are a million ways to be a runner. And although some ways work better than others from a performance standpoint, the runners who perform best over time tend to be those who, like Joan Benoit, give themselves permission to do it their way instead of blindly conforming to expectations. Certain rules can't be broken if you want to extend your peak years as a competitor. But within the framework defined by these unbreakable rules, there's plenty of freedom to find your own personal sweet spot, and the more stubborn independence you show in exercising this freedom, the better things will turn out for you.

DON'T LET YOURSELF GO

In the winter of 1987, when I was a junior in high school, I competed in an indoor track meet at Dartmouth College. Word got out during the meet that the legendary Henry Rono would be taking part in an open 5000 m race after the kids were finished competing. Already a huge fan of the sport, I knew all about Rono, who in 1978 had broken four world records at distances ranging from 3000 meters to 10,000 meters in the span of 81 days. Alcoholism soon derailed his career, but at age 34, Rono had committed himself to staging a comeback, and the indoor 5000 m race that I forced my entire team to hang around and watch instead of getting started on the long bus ride back home was his first rust buster.

It did not go well. Rono started out okay, pushing the pace up front with Jersey boy Marty Ludwikowski, but he never looked comfortable, and within a few laps, he'd begun to fall back. Having clocked 13:06 for the same distance 9 years earlier, he finished eighth in 14:38. His comeback fizzled not long thereafter.

Henry Rono's story is a cautionary tale for runners who want to run well not just today but also tomorrow and 10 years from now. It goes without saying that if you try to push hard all the time, you're not likely to perform at or near peak level for years on end. But longevity in the sport is just as unlikely if you back off too much, to the point of "letting yourself go," or dig yourself into a hole that's hard to get out of. Rono's alcoholism is an extreme example of the phenomenon, but there are less extreme and more common ways of letting oneself go that are also harmful to macropacing.

Take my brother Josh. Three years older than me, Josh started running at the same time I did, a few years before my close encounter with Henry Rono. We were closely matched in ability, our PBs only a few seconds apart at a variety of distances. But whereas I kept running throughout my twenties, thirties, and forties, Josh went for long stretches without ever lacing up his shoes and gained a lot of weight during these times. Consequently, when at age 48 he embarked on a quest to qualify for the Boston Marathon, it took him seemingly forever to excavate his talent from underneath the layers of disuse it was buried under. He got there eventually, but he often regretted those years of letting himself go.

I want to emphasize that the message here is not that you should never place running on life's back burner. Just be sure not to remove it from the stovetop entirely if you have any intention of racing well in the future.

STAY IN LOVE

Although I saved this fifth "rule" of macropacing for last, I think it's the most important one. If you spend time talking to a dozen runners who have succeeded in performing at or near their ultimate limit for a long time, the most striking shared quality you will see in them is a great passion for running. For proof, look no further than our friend Abdi Abdirahman, who told PodiumRunner's Hannah Borenstein before the 2020 Olympic Trials, "I love running. It's my hobby."

When an experienced runner continues to enjoy running year after year as much as they did when they first fell in love with the sport, they invariably find ways to keep running well. All too often, though, that initial thrill dissipates over time, and running becomes a mere habit maintained by its own inertia rather than by the force of passion. It's no tragedy for a runner to fall out of love with running and trade it for golf or rock climbing, but it is sad when a runner keeps putting the same amount of energy into their running as they did during the courting phase but no longer feels they're getting the same return in enjoyment.

When the thrill does fade, it does so typically because the runner forgets why they fell in love with running in the first place. In the beginning, it's running itself that brings joy, but all too often, as time passes, the act of putting one foot in front of the other becomes a means to an end—faster times, high-age-group finishes, hitting qualifying standards. The problem is that, for every goal a runner achieves, they complete hundreds of thousands of steps. So who do you think enjoys running more: the runner who achieves the occasional goal or the one who continues to find joy in the very act of running?

One runner who never forgot why he fell in love with running is Haile Gebrselassie. He started at age 7, inspired by the exploits of his older country-man Miruts Yifter, who won two gold medals for Ethiopia at the 1980 Olympics. Though his father discouraged the hobby, dismissing it as a waste of time, Geb ran anyway, a toothy smile expressing the pure bliss he felt as he traveled barefoot at 8,000 feet. That ever-present smile would become his trademark, inspiring one writer to describe him as "the happiest man in running."

I met Geb in 2009 at a press event hosted by his shoe sponsor in Los Angeles. Fresh off a victory at the Berlin Marathon, where he'd broken his own world record, he transformed an obligatory appearance into an unforgettable spectacle when he hijacked a demonstration of new Adidas gear by spontaneously running a 4-minute mile on a treadmill, beaming like a child on a playground. "A day without running is like a day without eating," he said in a 2013 interview for the *Guardian*. "I love running, and I will always run."

In a professional career that spanned nearly a quarter of a century, Haile Gebrselassie set an astonishing 27 world records and earned 9 Olympic and World Championship medals, 6 of them gold. Clearly, the childlike enthusiasm for running that he maintained from his first race till his last did not stop him from performing at his best. Quite the opposite, in fact. It is simply no accident that the person who loves running more than anyone else ever has and the most accomplished runner in history are the same person.

How to stay in love with running is no secret. It's just a matter of continuing to run for the same reason you did when you first fell in love, even as you make room in your heart for other reasons, such as achieving results. One thing that can help in this regard is checking in with yourself regularly about your relationship with running, perhaps through a journal. When you notice a dip in your enjoyment level, flag it and reflect on ways to rekindle the flame.

Most often, enjoyment dips when a runner becomes fixated on outcomes and rises when they focus on the moment-to-moment process. Relationship check-ins are just one way to do this. Others include self-reminder mantras such as the oldie but goodie, "Run the mile you're in." The main thing is to get in the habit of catching yourself in those moments when your mind tries to leap ahead to the endpoint so you can deploy whichever particular method is most appropriate for the situation.

To the extent that you succeed in shifting your focus from outcomes to the process, you will feel liberated, as though an invisible burden has been lifted from your shoulders. When you're focused on outcomes, you're essentially saying, "I will be happy if and only if I achieve my goal," a mindset that causes the quality of your running experience to depend on something over which you have only partial control. But when you're focused on the process, you're saying to yourself, "I'm going to enjoy doing my best in this run, win or lose," a mindset that puts you in total control of the quality of your experience.

Recently I attended a running camp where I met a runner named Traci, who had recently suffered through a disastrous first ultramarathon and was having trouble moving past it.

"What's the point?" she asked me rhetorically. "You train for months to achieve a goal, and then you fall flat on your face, and it all seems wasted."

"It sounds like you want a guarantee of success every time you start a race," I said. "But do you really? How much would success really mean if you couldn't fail?"

"I guess you're right," Traci conceded.

Lots of runners think they want guaranteed success, but there's very little satisfaction to be gleaned from a successful outcome when the true credit belongs not to the runner themselves but to some outside guarantee . . . or a sports watch. What runners like Traci really want is not guaranteed success but to be in control of their performance—to not need an omnipotent smartwatch or any other form of outside help to run a race they're proud of.

At the beginning of this book, I claimed that the most satisfying experience you can have as a competitive runner is knowing what you can do and then going out and doing it. The feeling of confident self-determination that comes with this knowledge makes the entire race experience enjoyable, regardless of outcome, and it is a feeling available only to those who master the skill of pacing at both levels, micro and macro—for this and only this can free a runner from all external dependencies.

A perfect race is not a race that goes perfectly. It's a race that the runner could not have completed any faster. The weather, good or bad, makes no difference. How you feel, good or bad, doesn't matter. A perfect race is achievable even when absolutely nothing goes your way. Success and failure are entirely within your control, depending on nothing else besides your capacity to read your body, to try really hard, and to make smart decisions. You might not have these capacities today, but I can assure you that the only way you will ever have them is by actively seeking them—something you now know how to do. Remember, a perfect race is a perfectly paced race, and pacing is the art of finding your limit. Don't wait for your limit to find you. It never will. Go find it!

9

5K Training Plans

The four training plans presented in this chapter are designed to help runners master the art of pacing and find their limit at the 5K distance. The various levels cover the needs of everyone from first-timers to elites. Refer back to Chapter 6 for details on the RPE-based intensity scale used throughout the plans and for full explanations of certain terms and workout types. Online versions of the plans are available for separate purchase on the 80/20 Endurance web site. Additionally, device-compatible free versions of the individual workouts can be found at https://www.8020endurance.com.

5K

This plan is appropriate for beginning runners preparing for their first 5K event and for more experienced runners who need or prefer a relatively low-volume training program for any reason. Before starting the plan, be sure to build your training to the point where you're comfortably able to run 5 days a week for up to 30 minutes.

	MONDAY	TUESDAY	WEDNESDAY	THURSDAY
1	Rest	**Fartleks** 5:00 at RPE 2–3 5:00 at RPE 3–4 6 × 0:20 at RPE 8–9 / 1:40 at RPE 2–3 10:00 at RPE 3–4	**Foundation Run** 5:00 at RPE 2–3 15:00 at RPE 3–4	Rest
2	Rest	**Fartleks** 5:00 at RPE 2–3 5:00 at RPE 3–4 4 × 1:00 at RPE 7–8 / 2:00 at RPE 2–3 10:00 at RPE 3–4	**Foundation Run** 5:00 at RPE 2–3 20:00 at RPE 3–4	Rest
3	Rest	**Hill Repetitions** 5:00 at RPE 2–3 5:00 at RPE 3–4 6 × 0:30* uphill at RPE 8–9 / 1:30 at RPE 2–3 10:00 at RPE 2–3 *Stretch Intervals*	**Foundation Run** 5:00 at RPE 2–3 20:00 at RPE 3–4	Rest
4	Rest	**VO₂max Intervals** 5:00 at RPE 2–3 5:00 at RPE 3–4 4 × 2:00* at RPE 7–8 / 1:00 at RPE 2–3 10:00 at RPE 2–3 *Precision Splitting*	**Foundation Run** 5:00 at RPE 2–3 25:00 at RPE 3–4	Rest
5	Rest	**Speed Intervals** 5:00 at RPE 2–3 5:00 at RPE 3–4 6 × 1:00* at RPE 8–9 / 2:00 at RPE 2–3 10:00 at RPE 2–3 *Stretch Intervals*	**Foundation Run** 5:00 at RPE 2–3 25:00 at RPE 3–4	Rest

How to Run the Perfect Race

LEVEL

SSP Steady-State Pace
LTP Lactate Threshold Pace
CV Critical Velocity
MAS Maximal Aerobic Speed

5K

FRIDAY	SATURDAY	SUNDAY
Progression Run 5:00 at RPE 2–3 10:00 at RPE 3–4 8:00 at SSP 4:00 at LTP 2:00 at CV 5:00 at RPE 2–3	**Foundation Run** 5:00 at RPE 2–3 15:00 at RPE 3–4	**Endurance Run** 5:00 at RPE 2–3 20:00 at RPE 3–4 5:00 at RPE 5–6
Progression Run 5:00 at RPE 2–3 20:00 at RPE 3–4 4:00 at LTP 2:00 at CV 1:00 at MAS 5:00 at RPE 2–3	**Foundation Run** 5:00 at RPE 2–3 20:00 at RPE 3–4	**Endurance Run** 5:00 at RPE 2–3 25:00 at RPE 3–4 5:00 at RPE 5–6
Fartleks 5:00 at RPE 2–3 5:00 at RPE 3–4 1:00 at CV, 1:00 at RPE 2–3 2:00 at LTP, 1:00 at RPE 2–3 3:00 at SSP, 1:00 at RPE 2–3 2:00 at LTP, 1:00 at RPE 2–3 1:00 at CV, 1:00 at RPE 2–3 10:00 at RPE 3–4	**Foundation Run** 5:00 at RPE 2–3 20:00 at RPE 3–4	**Endurance Run** 5:00 at RPE 2–3 20:00 at RPE 3–4 5:00 at RPE 5–6
Tempo Run 5:00 at RPE 2–3 5:00 at RPE 3–4 10:00 at RPE 6 5:00 at RPE 2–3 10:00 at RPE 6 10:00 at RPE 2–3	**Foundation Run** 5:00 at RPE 2–3 25:00 at RPE 3–4	**Endurance Run** 5:00 at RPE 2–3 30:00 at RPE 3–4 5:00 at RPE 5–6
Critical Velocity Intervals 5:00 at RPE 2–3 5:00 at RPE 3–4 4 × 4:00* at RPE 6–7 / 2:00 at RPE 2–3 10:00 at RPE 2–3 *Precision Splitting*	**Foundation Run** 5:00 at RPE 2–3 25:00 at RPE 3–4	**Endurance Run** 5:00 at RPE 2–3 35:00 at RPE 3–4 5:00 at RPE 5–6

	MONDAY	TUESDAY	WEDNESDAY	THURSDAY
6	Rest	**Accelerations** 5:00 at RPE 2–3 5:00 at RPE 3–4 11:00 acceleration 10:00 at RPE 2–3 3:00 acceleration 10:00 at RPE 2–3	**Foundation Run** 5:00 at RPE 2–3 25:00 at RPE 3–4	Rest
7	Rest	**VO_2max Intervals** 5:00 at RPE 2–3 5:00 at RPE 3–4 5 × 2:00* at RPE 7–8 / 1:00 at RPE 2–3 10:00 at RPE 2–3 **Precision Splitting*	**Foundation Run** 5:00 at RPE 2–3 30:00 at RPE 3–4	Rest
8	Rest	**Relaxed Time Trial** 1 km at RPE 2–3 1 km at RPE 3–4 5 km at 95% effort 1:00 rest 2 km at RPE 2–3	**Foundation Run** 5:00 at RPE 2–3 30:00 at RPE 3–4	Rest
9	Rest	**Fartleks** 5:00 at RPE 2–3 5:00 at RPE 3–4 6 × 1:00 at RPE 7–8 / 2:00 at RPE 2–3 10:00 at RPE 3–4	Rest	**Fast Finish Run** 5:00 at RPE 2–3 15:00 at RPE 3–4 5:00 at CV

FRIDAY	SATURDAY	SUNDAY
Progression Run 5:00 at RPE 2–3 25:00 at RPE 3–4 4:00 at LTP 2:00 at CV 1:00 at MAS 5:00 at RPE 2–3	**Foundation Run** 5:00 at RPE 2–3 25:00 at RPE 3–4	**Endurance Run** 5:00 at RPE 2–3 25:00 at RPE 3–4 5:00 at RPE 5–6
Tempo Run 5:00 at RPE 2–3 5:00 at RPE 3–4 12:00 at RPE 6 5:00 at RPE 2–3 12:00 at RPE 6 10:00 at RPE 2–3	**Foundation Run** 5:00 at RPE 2–3 30:00 at RPE 3–4	**Endurance Run** 5:00 at RPE 2–3 40:00 at RPE 3–4 5:00 at RPE 5–6
Critical Velocity Intervals 5:00 at RPE 2–3 5:00 at RPE 3–4 5 × 4:00* at RPE 6–7 / 2:00 at RPE 2–3 10:00 at RPE 2–3 *Precision Splitting*	**Foundation Run** 5:00 at RPE 2–3 30:00 at RPE 3–4	**Endurance Run** 5:00 at RPE 2–3 45:00 at RPE 3–4 5:00 at RPE 5–6
Foundation Run 5:00 at RPE 2–3 15:00 at RPE 3–4	**5K Race**	Rest

5K

This plan was designed for runners who are ready to take their training load up a notch in order to improve their 5K time. Before starting the plan, be sure to build your training to the point where you're comfortably able to run 6 days a week for up to 40 minutes.

	MONDAY	TUESDAY	WEDNESDAY	THURSDAY
1	Rest	**Fartleks** 5:00 at RPE 2–3 5:00 at RPE 3–4 6 × 0:20 at RPE 8–9 / 1:40 at RPE 2–3 10:00 at RPE 3–4	**Foundation Run** 5:00 at RPE 2–3 25:00 at RPE 3–4	**Foundation Run** 5:00 at RPE 2–3 25:00 at RPE 3–4
2	Rest	**Fartleks** 5:00 at RPE 2–3 5:00 at RPE 3–4 6 × 1:00 at RPE 7–8 / 2:00 at RPE 2–3 10:00 at RPE 3–4	**Foundation Run** 5:00 at RPE 2–3 25:00 at RPE 3–4	**Foundation Run** 5:00 at RPE 2–3 25:00 at RPE 3–4
3	Rest	**Hill Repetitions** 5:00 at RPE 2–3 5:00 at RPE 3–4 6 × 0:30* uphill at RPE 8–9 / 1:30 at RPE 2–3 10:00 at RPE 2–3 *Stretch Intervals*	**Foundation Run** 5:00 at RPE 2–3 25:00 at RPE 3–4	**Foundation Run** 5:00 at RPE 2–3 25:00 at RPE 3–4
4	Rest	**VO$_2$max Intervals** 5:00 at RPE 2–3 5:00 at RPE 3–4 4 × 2:00* at RPE 7–8 / 1:00 at RPE 2–3 10:00 at RPE 2–3 *Precision Splitting*	**Foundation Run** 5:00 at RPE 2–3 30:00 at RPE 3–4	**Foundation Run** 5:00 at RPE 2–3 30:00 at RPE 3–4
5	Rest	**Speed Intervals** 5:00 at RPE 2–3 5:00 at RPE 3–4 7 × 1:00* at RPE 8–9 / 2:00 at RPE 2–3 10:00 at RPE 2–3 *Stretch Intervals*	**Foundation Run** 5:00 at RPE 2–3 30:00 at RPE 3–4	**Foundation Run** 5:00 at RPE 2–3 30:00 at RPE 3–4

LEVEL

SSP Steady-State Pace
LTP Lactate Threshold Pace
CV Critical Velocity
MAS Maximal Aerobic Speed

FRIDAY	SATURDAY	SUNDAY
Progression Run 5:00 at RPE 2–3 25:00 at RPE 3–4 4:00 at LTP 2:00 at CV 1:00 at MAS 5:00 at RPE 2–3	**Foundation Run** 5:00 at RPE 2–3 25:00 at RPE 3–4	**Endurance Run** 5:00 at RPE 2–3 30:00 at RPE 3–4 5:00 at RPE 5–6
Progression Run 5:00 at RPE 2–3 20:00 at RPE 3–4 8:00 at SSP 4:00 at LTP 2:00 at CV 5:00 at RPE 2–3	**Foundation Run** 5:00 at RPE 2–3 25:00 at RPE 3–4	**Endurance Run** 5:00 at RPE 2–3 40:00 at RPE 3–4 5:00 at RPE 5–6
Fartleks 5:00 at RPE 2–3 5:00 at RPE 3–4 1:00 at CV, 1:00 at RPE 2–3 2:00 at LTP, 1:00 at RPE 2–3 3:00 at SSP, 1:00 at RPE 2–3 2:00 at LTP, 1:00 at RPE 2–3 1:00 at CV, 1:00 at RPE 2–3 10:00 at RPE 3–4	**Foundation Run** 5:00 at RPE 2–3 25:00 at RPE 3–4	**Endurance Run** 5:00 at RPE 2–3 30:00 at RPE 3–4 5:00 at RPE 5–6
Tempo Run 5:00 at RPE 2–3 5:00 at RPE 3–4 10:00 at RPE 6 5:00 at RPE 2–3 10:00 at RPE 6 10:00 at RPE 2–3	**Foundation Run** 5:00 at RPE 2–3 30:00 at RPE 3–4	**Endurance Run** 5:00 at RPE 2–3 50:00 at RPE 3–4 5:00 at RPE 5–6
Critical Velocity Intervals 5:00 at RPE 2–3 5:00 at RPE 3–4 4 × 4:00* at RPE 6–7 / 2:00 at RPE 2–3 10:00 at RPE 2–3 *Precision Splitting*	**Foundation Run** 5:00 at RPE 2–3 30:00 at RPE 3–4	**Endurance Run** 5:00 at RPE 2–3 1:00:00 at RPE 3–4 5:00 at RPE 5–6

	MONDAY	TUESDAY	WEDNESDAY	THURSDAY
6	Rest	**Accelerations** 5:00 at RPE 2–3 5:00 at RPE 3–4 11:00 acceleration 10:00 at RPE 2–3 3:00 acceleration 10:00 at RPE 2–3	**Foundation Run** 5:00 at RPE 2–3 25:00 at RPE 3–4	**Foundation Run** 5:00 at RPE 2–3 25:00 at RPE 3–4
7	Rest	**The Prefontaine** 1 km at RPE 2–3 1 km at RPE 3–4 ? × 200m at RPE 9 / 200m at RPE 6 1 km at RPE 2–3 1 km at RPE 3–4 *(? = Go to failure)*	**Foundation Run** 5:00 at RPE 2–3 35:00 at RPE 3–4	**Foundation Run** 5:00 at RPE 2–3 35:00 at RPE 3–4
8	Rest	**Relaxed Time Trial** 1 km at RPE 2–3 1 km at RPE 3–4 5 km at 95% effort 1:00 rest 2 km at RPE 2–3	**Foundation Run** 5:00 at RPE 2–3 35:00 at RPE 3–4	**Foundation Run** 5:00 at RPE 2–3 35:00 at RPE 3–4
9	Rest	**Fartleks** 5:00 at RPE 2–3 5:00 at RPE 3–4 8 × 1:00 at RPE 7–8 / 2:00 at RPE 2–3 10:00 at RPE 3–4	**Foundation Run** 5:00 at RPE 2–3 30:00 at RPE 3–4	**Fast Finish Run** 5:00 at RPE 2–3 20:00 at RPE 3–4 5:00 at CV

FRIDAY	SATURDAY	SUNDAY
Progression Run 5:00 at RPE 2–3 25:00 at RPE 3–4 4:00 at LTP 2:00 at CV 1:00 at MAS 5:00 at RPE 2–3	**Foundation Run** 5:00 at RPE 2–3 25:00 at RPE 3–4	**Endurance Run** 5:00 at RPE 2–3 40:00 at RPE 3–4 5:00 at RPE 5–6
Tempo Run 5:00 at RPE 2–3 5:00 at RPE 3–4 12:00 at RPE 6 5:00 at RPE 2–3 12:00 at RPE 6 10:00 at RPE 2–3	**Foundation Run** 5:00 at RPE 2–3 35:00 at RPE 3–4	**Endurance Run** 5:00 at RPE 2–3 1:10:00 at RPE 3–4 5:00 at RPE 5–6
Critical Velocity Intervals 5:00 at RPE 2–3 5:00 at RPE 3–4 5 × 4:00* at RPE 6–7 / 2:00 at RPE 2–3 10:00 at RPE 2–3 *Precision Splitting*	**Foundation Run** 5:00 at RPE 2–3 35:00 at RPE 3–4	**Endurance Run** 5:00 at RPE 2–3 50:00 at RPE 3–4 5:00 at RPE 5–6
Foundation Run 5:00 at RPE 2–3 15:00 at RPE 3–4	**5K Race**	Rest

5K

This plan is a good fit for experienced competitive runners who are prepared to train hard in pursuit of improved 5K performance. Before starting the plan, be sure to build your training to the point where you're comfortably able to run 7 days a week for up to 70 minutes.

	MONDAY	TUESDAY	WEDNESDAY	THURSDAY
1	**Recovery Run** 30:00 at RPE 2–3	**Fartleks** 5:00 at RPE 2–3 10:00 at RPE 3–4 8 × 0:20 at RPE 8–9 / 1:40 at RPE 2–3 15:00 at RPE 3–4	**Foundation Run** 5:00 at RPE 2–3 35:00 at RPE 3–4	**Foundation Run** 5:00 at RPE 2–3 55:00 at RPE 3–4
2	**Recovery Run** 30:00 at RPE 2–3	**Fartleks** 5:00 at RPE 2–3 10:00 at RPE 3–4 8 × 1:00 at RPE 7–8 / 2:00 at RPE 2–3 15:00 at RPE 3–4	**Foundation Run** 5:00 at RPE 2–3 35:00 at RPE 3–4	**Foundation Run** 5:00 at RPE 2–3 55:00 at RPE 3–4
3	Rest	**Hill Repetitions** 5:00 at RPE 2–3 10:00 at RPE 3–4 8 × 0:30* uphill at RPE 8–9 / 1:30 at RPE 2–3 15:00 at RPE 2–3 *Stretch Intervals*	**Foundation Run** 5:00 at RPE 2–3 35:00 at RPE 3–4	**Foundation Run** 5:00 at RPE 2–3 55:00 at RPE 3–4
4	**Recovery Run** 30:00 at RPE 2–3	**VO$_2$max Intervals** 5:00 at RPE 2–3 10:00 at RPE 3–4 5 × 2:00* at RPE 7–8 / 1:00 at RPE 2–3 15:00 at RPE 2–3 *Precision Splitting*	**Foundation Run** 5:00 at RPE 2–3 40:00 at RPE 3–4	**Foundation Run** 5:00 at RPE 2–3 55:00 at RPE 3–4

How to Run the Perfect Race

LEVEL

SSP Steady-State Pace
LTP Lactate Threshold Pace
CV Critical Velocity
MAS Maximal Aerobic Speed

10KP 10K Pace

FRIDAY	SATURDAY	SUNDAY
Progression Run 5:00 at RPE 2–3 30:00 at RPE 3–4 4:00 at LTP 2:00 at CV 1:00 at MAS 5:00 at RPE 2–3	**Foundation Run** 5:00 at RPE 2–3 35:00 at RPE 3–4	**Endurance Run** 5:00 at RPE 2–3 1:00:00 at RPE 3–4 5:00 at RPE 5–6
Progression Run 5:00 at RPE 2–3 30:00 at RPE 3–4 8:00 at SSP 4:00 at LTP 2:00 at CV 5:00 at RPE 2–3	**Foundation Run** 5:00 at RPE 2–3 35:00 at RPE 3–4	**Steady-State Run** 5:00 at RPE 2–3 10:00 at RPE 3–4 30:00 at RPE 5 15:00 at RPE 2–3
Fartleks 5:00 at RPE 2–3 10:00 at RPE 3–4 1:00 at CV, 1:00 at RPE 2–3 2:00 at LTP, 1:00 at RPE 2–3 3:00 at SSP, 1:00 at RPE 2–3 2:00 at LTP, 1:00 at RPE 2–3 1:00 at CV, 1:00 at RPE 2–3 15:00 at RPE 3–4	**Foundation Run** 5:00 at RPE 2–3 35:00 at RPE 3–4	**Endurance Run** 5:00 at RPE 2–3 1:10:00 at RPE 3–4 5:00 at RPE 5–6
Critical Velocity Intervals 5:00 at RPE 2–3 10:00 at RPE 3–4 5 × 4:00* at RPE 6–7 / 2:00 at RPE 2–3 15:00 at RPE 2–3 *Precision Splitting*	**Foundation Run** 5:00 at RPE 2–3 40:00 at RPE 3–4	**Tempo Run** 5:00 at RPE 2–3 10:00 at RPE 3–4 8:00 at RPE 6 5:00 at RPE 2–3 8:00 at RPE 6 5:00 at RPE 2–3 8:00 at RPE 6 15:00 at RPE 2–3

5K

2

	MONDAY	TUESDAY	WEDNESDAY	THURSDAY
5	**Recovery Run** 30:00 at RPE 2–3	**Relaxed Time Trial** 1 km at RPE 2–3 2 km at RPE 3–4 5 km at 95% effort 1:00 rest 3 km at RPE 2–3	**Foundation Run** 5:00 at RPE 2–3 40:00 at RPE 3–4	**Foundation Run** 5:00 at RPE 2–3 55:00 at RPE 3–4
6	Rest	**Accelerations** 5:00 at RPE 2–3 10:00 at RPE 3–4 11:00 acceleration 10:00 at RPE 2–3 6:00 acceleration 15:00 at RPE 2–3	**Foundation Run** 5:00 at RPE 2–3 35:00 at RPE 3–4	**Foundation Run** 5:00 at RPE 2–3 55:00 at RPE 3–4
7	**Recovery Run** 30:00 at RPE 2–3	**The Prefontaine** 1 km at RPE 2–3 2.5 km at RPE 3–4 ? × 200m at RPE 9 / 200m at RPE 6 1 km at RPE 2–3 2.5 km at RPE 3–4 *(? = Go to failure)*	**Foundation Run** 5:00 at RPE 2–3 45:00 at RPE 3–4	**Foundation Run** 5:00 at RPE 2–3 55:00 at RPE 3–4
8	**Recovery Run** 30:00 at RPE 2–3	**5K Pace Intervals** 1 km at RPE 2–3 2 km at RPE 3–4 6 × (0.8 km at 10KP / 1:00 rest) 3 km at RPE 2–3	**Foundation Run** 5:00 at RPE 2–3 45:00 at RPE 3–4	**Foundation Run** 5:00 at RPE 2–3 55:00 at RPE 3–4
9	Rest	**Speed Intervals** 5:00 at RPE 2–3 10:00 at RPE 3–4 10 × 0:30* at RPE 8–9 / 1:30 at RPE 2–3 15:00 at RPE 2–3 **Stretch Intervals*	**Foundation Run** 5:00 at RPE 2–3 35:00 at RPE 3–4	**Fast Finish Run** 5:00 at RPE 2–3 25:00 at RPE 3–4 5:00 at CV

FRIDAY	SATURDAY	SUNDAY
Speed Intervals 5:00 at RPE 2–3 10:00 at RPE 3–4 10 × 1:00* at RPE 8–9 / 　2:00 at RPE 2–3 15:00 at RPE 2–3 *Stretch Intervals*	**Foundation Run** 5:00 at RPE 2–3 40:00 at RPE 3–4	**Steady-State Run** 5:00 at RPE 2–3 10:00 at RPE 3–4 35:00 at RPE 5 15:00 at RPE 2–3
Progression Run 5:00 at RPE 2–3 35:00 at RPE 3–4 4:00 at LTP 2:00 at CV 1:00 at MAS 5:00 at RPE 2–3	**Foundation Run** 5:00 at RPE 2–3 35:00 at RPE 3–4	**Endurance Run** 5:00 at RPE 2–3 1:20:00 at RPE 3–4 5:00 at RPE 5–6
10K Pace Intervals 1 km at RPE 2–3 2 km at RPE 3–4 8 × (1 km at 10KP / 1:00 rest) 3 km at RPE 2–3	**Foundation Run** 5:00 at RPE 2–3 45:00 at RPE 3–4	**Tempo Run** 5:00 at RPE 2–3 10:00 at RPE 3–4 10:00 at RPE 6 5:00 at RPE 2–3 10:00 at RPE 6 5:00 at RPE 2–3 10:00 at RPE 6 15:00 at RPE 2–3
Critical Velocity Intervals 5:00 at RPE 2–3 10:00 at RPE 3–4 6 × 4:00* at RPE 6–7 / 　2:00 at RPE 2–3 15:00 at RPE 2–3 *Precision Splitting*	**Foundation Run** 5:00 at RPE 2–3 45:00 at RPE 3–4	**Progression Run** 5:00 at RPE 2–3 25:00 at RPE 3–4 16:00 at SSP 8:00 at LTP 4:00 at CV 5:00 at RPE 2–3
Foundation Run 5:00 at RPE 2–3 15:00 at RPE 3–4	**5K Race**	Rest

5K

This plan is designed for serious, competitive runners seeking the absolute limit of their potential at the 5K distance. Before starting the plan, be sure to build your training to the point where you're comfortably able to run 9 times a week for up to 80 minutes.

	MONDAY	TUESDAY	WEDNESDAY	THURSDAY
1	**Recovery Run** 40:00 at RPE 2–3	**Fartleks** 5:00 at RPE 2–3 15:00 at RPE 3–4 10 × 0:20 at RPE 8–9 / 1:40 at RPE 2–3 20:00 at RPE 3–4 **Recovery Run** 20:00 at RPE 2–3	**Foundation Run** 5:00 at RPE 2–3 40:00 at RPE 3–4	**Foundation Run** 5:00 at RPE 2–3 55:00 at RPE 3–4
2	**Recovery Run** 40:00 at RPE 2–3	**Fartleks** 5:00 at RPE 2–3 15:00 at RPE 3–4 10 × 1:00 at RPE 7–8 / 2:00 at RPE 2–3 20:00 at RPE 3–4 **Recovery Run** 20:00 at RPE 2–3	**Foundation Run** 5:00 at RPE 2–3 45:00 at RPE 3–4	**Foundation Run** 5:00 at RPE 2–3 55:00 at RPE 3–4
3	Rest	**Hill Repetitions** 5:00 at RPE 2–3 15:00 at RPE 3–4 10 × 0:30* uphill at RPE 8–9 / 1:30 at RPE 2–3 20:00 at RPE 2–3 *Stretch Intervals **Recovery Run** 20:00 at RPE 2–3	**Foundation Run** 5:00 at RPE 2–3 40:00 at RPE 3–4	**Foundation Run** 5:00 at RPE 2–3 55:00 at RPE 3–4

LEVEL

SSP Steady-State Pace
LTP Lactate Threshold Pace
CV Critical Velocity
MAS Maximal Aerobic Speed

10KP 10K Pace

FRIDAY	SATURDAY	SUNDAY
Progression Run 5:00 at RPE 2–3 35:00 at RPE 3–4 4:00 at LTP 2:00 at CV 1:00 at MAS 5:00 at RPE 2–3 **Recovery Run** 20:00 at RPE 2–3	**Foundation Run** 5:00 at RPE 2–3 40:00 at RPE 3–4	**Endurance Run** 5:00 at RPE 2–3 1:10:00 at RPE 3–4 5:00 at RPE 5–6
Progression Run 5:00 at RPE 2–3 25:00 at RPE 3–4 12:00 at SSP 6:00 at LTP 3:00 at CV 5:00 at RPE 2–3 **Recovery Run** 20:00 at RPE 2–3	**Foundation Run** 5:00 at RPE 2–3 45:00 at RPE 3–4	**Steady-State Run** 5:00 at RPE 2–3 15:00 at RPE 3–4 35:00 at RPE 5 20:00 at RPE 2–3
Fartleks 5:00 at RPE 2–3 15:00 at RPE 3–4 1:00 at CV, 1:00 at RPE 2–3 2:00 at LTP, 1:00 at RPE 2–3 3:00 at SSP, 1:00 at RPE 2–3 2:00 at LTP, 1:00 at RPE 2–3 1:00 at CV, 1:00 at RPE 2–3 2:00 at LTP, 1:00 at RPE 2–3 3:00 at SSP 20:00 at RPE 3–4 **Recovery Run** 20:00 at RPE 2–3	**Foundation Run** 5:00 at RPE 2–3 40:00 at RPE 3–4	**Endurance Run** 5:00 at RPE 2–3 1:30:00 at RPE 3–4 5:00 at RPE 5–6

3 5K

	MONDAY	TUESDAY	WEDNESDAY	THURSDAY
4	**Recovery Run** 40:00 at RPE 2–3	**VO$_2$max Intervals** 5:00 at RPE 2–3 15:00 at RPE 3–4 6 × 2:00* at RPE 7–8 / 1:00 at RPE 2–3 20:00 at RPE 2–3 *Precision Splitting* **Recovery Run** 25:00 at RPE 2–3	**Foundation Run** 5:00 at RPE 2–3 50:00 at RPE 3–4	**Foundation Run** 5:00 at RPE 2–3 55:00 at RPE 3–4
5	**Recovery Run** 40:00 at RPE 2–3	**Relaxed Time Trial** 1 km at RPE 2–3 3 km at RPE 3–4 5 km at 95% effort 1:00 rest 4 km at RPE 2–3 **Recovery Run** 25:00 at RPE 2–3	**Foundation Run** 5:00 at RPE 2–3 55:00 at RPE 3–4	**Foundation Run** 5:00 at RPE 2–3 55:00 at RPE 3–4
6	Rest	**Accelerations** 5:00 at RPE 2–3 15:00 at RPE 3–4 11:00 acceleration 10:00 at RPE 2–3 6:00 acceleration 20:00 at RPE 2–3 **Recovery Run** 20:00 at RPE 2–3	**Foundation Run** 5:00 at RPE 2–3 45:00 at RPE 3–4	**Foundation Run** 5:00 at RPE 2–3 55:00 at RPE 3–4
7	**Recovery Run** 40:00 at RPE 2–3	**The Prefontaine** 1 km at RPE 2–3 4 km at RPE 3–4 ? × 200m at RPE 9 / 200m at RPE 6 1 km at RPE 2–3 4 km at RPE 3–4 *(? = Go to failure)* **Recovery Run** 30:00 at RPE 2–3	**Foundation Run** 5:00 at RPE 2–3 55:00 at RPE 3–4	**Foundation Run** 5:00 at RPE 2–3 1:00:00 at RPE 3–4
8	**Recovery Run** 40:00 at RPE 2–3	**5K Pace Intervals** 1 km at RPE 2–3 2 km at RPE 3–4 6 × (0.8 km at 10KP / 1:00 rest) 3 km at RPE 2–3 **Recovery Run** 30:00 at RPE 2–3	**Foundation Run** 5:00 at RPE 2–3 55:00 at RPE 3–4	**Foundation Run** 5:00 at RPE 2–3 1:05:00 at RPE 3–4
9	Rest	**Speed Intervals** 5:00 at RPE 2–3 15:00 at RPE 3–4 10 × 0:30* at RPE 8–9 / 1:30 at RPE 2–3 20:00 at RPE 2–3 *Stretch Intervals*	**Foundation Run** 5:00 at RPE 2–3 55:00 at RPE 3–4	**Fast Finish Run** 5:00 at RPE 2–3 30:00 at RPE 3–4 5:00 at CV

FRIDAY	SATURDAY	SUNDAY
Critical Velocity Intervals 5:00 at RPE 2–3 15:00 at RPE 3–4 6 × 4:00* at RPE 6–7 / 2:00 at RPE 2–3 20:00 at RPE 2–3 *Precision Splitting* **Recovery Run** 25:00 at RPE 2–3	**Foundation Run** 5:00 at RPE 2–3 50:00 at RPE 3–4	**Tempo Run** 5:00 at RPE 2–3 15:00 at RPE 3–4 10:00 at RPE 6 5:00 at RPE 2–3 10:00 at RPE 6 5:00 at RPE 2–3 10:00 at RPE 6 20:00 at RPE 2–3
Speed Intervals 5:00 at RPE 2–3 15:00 at RPE 3–4 12 × 1:00* at RPE 8–9 / 2:00 at RPE 2–3 20:00 at RPE 2–3 *Stretch Intervals* **Recovery Run** 25:00 at RPE 2–3	**Foundation Run** 5:00 at RPE 2–3 55:00 at RPE 3–4	**Steady-State Run** 5:00 at RPE 2–3 15:00 at RPE 3–4 40:00 at RPE 5 20:00 at RPE 2–3
Progression Run 5:00 at RPE 2–3 30:00 at RPE 3–4 8:00 at LTP 4:00 at CV 2:00 at MAS 5:00 at RPE 2–3 **Recovery Run** 20:00 at RPE 2–3	**Foundation Run** 5:00 at RPE 2–3 45:00 at RPE 3–4	**Endurance Run** 5:00 at RPE 2–3 1:50:00 at RPE 3–4 5:00 at RPE 5–6
10K Pace Intervals 1 km at RPE 2–3 3 km at RPE 3–4 8 × (1 km at 10KP / 1:00 rest) 4 km at RPE 2–3 **Recovery Run** 30:00 at RPE 2–3	**Foundation Run** 5:00 at RPE 2–3 55:00 at RPE 3–4	**Tempo Run** 5:00 at RPE 2–3 15:00 at RPE 3–4 12:00 at RPE 6 5:00 at RPE 2–3 12:00 at RPE 6 5:00 at RPE 2–3 12:00 at RPE 6 20:00 at RPE 2–3
Critical Velocity Intervals 5:00 at RPE 2–3 10:00 at RPE 3–4 6 × 4:00* at RPE 6–7 / 2:00 at RPE 2–3 15:00 at RPE 2–3 *Precision Splitting* **Recovery Run** 30:00 at RPE 2–3	**Foundation Run** 5:00 at RPE 2–3 55:00 at RPE 3–4	**Progression Run** 5:00 at RPE 2–3 35:00 at RPE 3–4 16:00 at SSP 8:00 at LTP 4:00 at CV 5:00 at RPE 2–3
Foundation Run 5:00 at RPE 2–3 15:00 at RPE 3–4	**5K Race**	Rest

10

10K Training Plans

The four training plans presented in this chapter are designed to help runners master the art of pacing and find their limit at the 10K distance. The various levels cover the needs of everyone from first-timers to elites. Refer back to Chapter 6 for details on the RPE-based intensity scale used throughout the plans and for full explanations of certain terms and workout types. Online versions of the plans are available for separate purchase on the 80/20 Endurance web site. Additionally, device-compatible free versions of the individual workouts can be found at https://www.8020endurance.com.

10K

This plan is appropriate for beginning runners preparing for their first 10K event and for more experienced runners who need or prefer a relatively low-volume training program for any reason. Before starting the plan, be sure to build your training to the point where you're comfortably able to run 5 days a week for up to 40 minutes.

	MONDAY	TUESDAY	WEDNESDAY	THURSDAY
1	Rest	**Fartleks** 5:00 at RPE 2–3 5:00 at RPE 3–4 6 × 0:20 at RPE 8–9 / 1:40 at RPE 2–3 10:00 at RPE 3–4	**Foundation Run** 5:00 at RPE 2–3 20:00 at RPE 3–4	Rest
2	Rest	**Fartleks** 5:00 at RPE 2–3 5:00 at RPE 3–4 6 × 1:00 at RPE 7–8 / 2:00 at RPE 2–3 10:00 at RPE 3–4	**Foundation Run** 5:00 at RPE 2–3 20:00 at RPE 3–4	Rest
3	Rest	**Hill Repetitions** 5:00 at RPE 2–3 5:00 at RPE 3–4 6 × 0:30 uphill at RPE 8–9 / 1:30 at RPE 2–3 10:00 at RPE 2–3	**Foundation Run** 5:00 at RPE 2–3 20:00 at RPE 3–4	Rest
4	Rest	**VO₂max Intervals** 5:00 at RPE 2–3 5:00 at RPE 3–4 4 × 2:00 at RPE 7–8 / 1:00 at RPE 2–3 10:00 at RPE 2–3	**Foundation Run** 5:00 at RPE 2–3 25:00 at RPE 3–4	Rest
5	Rest	**Accelerations** 5:00 at RPE 2–3 5:00 at RPE 3–4 11:00 acceleration 10:00 at RPE 2–3 3:00 acceleration 10:00 at RPE 2–3	**Foundation Run** 5:00 at RPE 2–3 25:00 at RPE 3–4	Rest

LEVEL

SSP Steady-State Pace
LTP Lactate Threshold Pace
CV Critical Velocity
MAS Maximal Aerobic Speed

5KP 5K Pace
10KP 10K Pace

FRIDAY	SATURDAY	SUNDAY
Progression Run 5:00 at RPE 2–3 10:00 at RPE 3–4 8:00 at SSP 4:00 at LTP 2:00 at CV 5:00 at RPE 2–3	**Foundation Run** 5:00 at RPE 2–3 20:00 at RPE 3–4	**Endurance Run** 5:00 at RPE 2–3 30:00 at RPE 3–4 5:00 at RPE 4–5
Progression Run 5:00 at RPE 2–3 20:00 at RPE 3–4 4:00 at LTP 2:00 at CV 1:00 at MAS 5:00 at RPE 2–3	**Foundation Run** 5:00 at RPE 2–3 20:00 at RPE 3–4	**Endurance Run** 5:00 at RPE 2–3 35:00 at RPE 3–4 5:00 at RPE 4–5
Fartleks 5:00 at RPE 2–3 5:00 at RPE 3–4 1:00 at CV, 1:00 at RPE 2–3 2:00 at LTP, 1:00 at RPE 2–3 3:00 at SSP, 1:00 at RPE 2–3 2:00 at LTP, 1:00 at RPE 2–3 1:00 at CV, 1:00 at RPE 2–3 10:00 at RPE 3–4	**Foundation Run** 5:00 at RPE 2–3 20:00 at RPE 3–4	**Endurance Run** 5:00 at RPE 2–3 30:00 at RPE 3–4 5:00 at RPE 4–5
Tempo Run 5:00 at RPE 2–3 5:00 at RPE 3–4 10:00 at RPE 6 5:00 at RPE 2–3 10:00 at RPE 6 10:00 at RPE 2–3	**Foundation Run** 5:00 at RPE 2–3 25:00 at RPE 3–4	**Endurance Run** 5:00 at RPE 2–3 40:00 at RPE 3–4 5:00 at RPE 4–5
Critical Velocity Intervals 5:00 at RPE 2–3 5:00 at RPE 3–4 4 × 4:00 at RPE 6–7 / 2:00 at RPE 2–3 10:00 at RPE 2–3	**Foundation Run** 5:00 at RPE 2–3 25:00 at RPE 3–4	**Endurance Run** 5:00 at RPE 2–3 45:00 at RPE 3–4 5:00 at RPE 4–5

	MONDAY	TUESDAY	WEDNESDAY	THURSDAY
6	Rest	**Hill Repetitions** 5:00 at RPE 2–3 5:00 at RPE 3–4 8 × 0:30 uphill at RPE 8–9 / 1:30 at RPE 2–3 10:00 at RPE 2–3	**Foundation Run** 5:00 at RPE 2–3 25:00 at RPE 3–4	Rest
7	Rest	**5K Pace Intervals** 1 km at RPE 2–3 1 km at RPE 3–4 8 × (0.6 km at 5KP / 1:00 rest) 2 km at RPE 2–3	**Foundation Run** 5:00 at RPE 2–3 30:00 at RPE 3–4	Rest
8	Rest	**Speed Intervals** 5:00 at RPE 2–3 5:00 at RPE 3–4 8 × 0:45 at RPE 8–9 / 1:45 at RPE 2–3 10:00 at RPE 2–3	**Foundation Run** 5:00 at RPE 2–3 30:00 at RPE 3–4	Rest
9	Rest	**Accelerations** 5:00 at RPE 2–3 5:00 at RPE 3–4 11:00 acceleration 10:00 at RPE 2–3 6:00 acceleration 10:00 at RPE 2–3	**Foundation Run** 5:00 at RPE 2–3 30:00 at RPE 3–4	Rest
10	Rest	**VO$_2$max Intervals** 5:00 at RPE 2–3 5:00 at RPE 3–4 5 × 2:00 at RPE 7–8 / 1:00 at RPE 2–3 10:00 at RPE 2–3	**Foundation Run** 5:00 at RPE 2–3 35:00 at RPE 3–4	Rest
11	Rest	**5K Pace Intervals** 1 km at RPE 2–3 1 km at RPE 3–4 6 × (0.8 km at 5KP / 1:00 rest) 2 km at RPE 2–3	**Foundation Run** 5:00 at RPE 2–3 35:00 at RPE 3–4	Rest
12	Rest	**Fartleks** 5:00 at RPE 2–3 5:00 at RPE 3–4 6 × 1:00 at RPE 7–8 / 2:00 at RPE 2–3 10:00 at RPE 3–4	Rest	**Fast Finish Run** 5:00 at RPE 2–3 10:00 at RPE 3–4 5:00 at RPE 6–7

FRIDAY	SATURDAY	SUNDAY
Progression Run 5:00 at RPE 2–3 10:00 at RPE 3–4 12:00 at SSP 6:00 at LTP 3:00 at CV 5:00 at RPE 2–3	**Foundation Run** 5:00 at RPE 2–3 25:00 at RPE 3–4	**Endurance Run** 5:00 at RPE 2–3 35:00 at RPE 3–4 5:00 at RPE 4–5
Steady-State Run 5:00 at RPE 2–3 5:00 at RPE 3–4 25:00 at RPE 5 10:00 at RPE 2–3	**Foundation Run** 5:00 at RPE 2–3 30:00 at RPE 3–4	**Endurance Run** 5:00 at RPE 2–3 50:00 at RPE 3–4 5:00 at RPE 4–5
Tempo Run 5:00 at RPE 2–3 5:00 at RPE 3–4 12:00 at RPE 6 5:00 at RPE 2–3 12:00 at RPE 6 10:00 at RPE 2–3	**Foundation Run** 5:00 at RPE 2–3 30:00 at RPE 3–4	**Endurance Run** 5:00 at RPE 2–3 1:00:00 at RPE 3–4 5:00 at RPE 4–5
Fartleks 5:00 at RPE 2–3 5:00 at RPE 3–4 1:00 at CV, 1:00 at RPE 2–3 2:00 at LTP, 1:00 at RPE 2–3 3:00 at SSP, 1:00 at RPE 2–3 2:00 at LTP, 1:00 at RPE 2–3 1:00 at CV, 1:00 at RPE 2–3 2:00 at LTP, 1:00 at RPE 2–3 3:00 at SSP, 1:00 at RPE 2–3 10:00 at RPE 3–4	**Foundation Run** 5:00 at RPE 2–3 30:00 at RPE 3–4	**Endurance Run** 5:00 at RPE 2–3 40:00 at RPE 3–4 5:00 at RPE 4–5
Critical Velocity Intervals 5:00 at RPE 2–3 5:00 at RPE 3–4 5 × 4:00 at RPE 6–7 / 2:00 at RPE 2–3 10:00 at RPE 2–3	**Foundation Run** 5:00 at RPE 2–3 35:00 at RPE 3–4	**Endurance Run** 5:00 at RPE 2–3 1:10:00 at RPE 3–4 5:00 at RPE 4–5
Fartleks 5:00 at RPE 2–3 5:00 at RPE 3–4 6 × 2:00 at RPE 6 / 2:00 at RPE 2–3 10:00 at RPE 3–4	**Foundation Run** 5:00 at RPE 2–3 35:00 at RPE 3–4	**10K Pace Intervals** 1 km at RPE 2–3 2 km at RPE 3–4 8 × (1 km at 10KP / 1:00 rest) 3 km at RPE 2–3
Foundation Run 5:00 at RPE 2–3 15:00 at RPE 3–4	**10K Race**	Rest

10K

O

10K

This plan is designed for runners who are ready to take their training load up a notch in order to improve their 10K time. Before starting the plan, be sure to build your training to the point where you're comfortably able to run 6 days a week for up to 40 minutes.

	MONDAY	TUESDAY	WEDNESDAY	THURSDAY
1	Rest	**Fartleks** 5:00 at RPE 2–3 5:00 at RPE 3–4 8 × 0:20 at RPE 8–9 / 1:40 at RPE 2–3 10:00 at RPE 3–4	**Foundation Run** 5:00 at RPE 2–3 25:00 at RPE 3–4	**Foundation Run** 5:00 at RPE 2–3 25:00 at RPE 3–4
2	Rest	**Fartleks** 5:00 at RPE 2–3 5:00 at RPE 3–4 8 × 1:00 at RPE 7–8 / 2:00 at RPE 2–3 10:00 at RPE 3–4	**Foundation Run** 5:00 at RPE 2–3 25:00 at RPE 3–4	**Foundation Run** 5:00 at RPE 2–3 25:00 at RPE 3–4
3	Rest	**Hill Repetitions** 5:00 at RPE 2–3 5:00 at RPE 3–4 8 × 0:30 uphill at RPE 8–9 / 1:30 at RPE 2–3 10:00 at RPE 2–3	**Foundation Run** 5:00 at RPE 2–3 25:00 at RPE 3–4	**Foundation Run** 5:00 at RPE 2–3 25:00 at RPE 3–4
4	Rest	**VO$_2$max Intervals** 5:00 at RPE 2–3 5:00 at RPE 3–4 5 × 2:00 at RPE 7–8 / 1:00 at RPE 2–3 10:00 at RPE 2–3	**Foundation Run** 5:00 at RPE 2–3 30:00 at RPE 3–4	**Foundation Run** 5:00 at RPE 2–3 30:00 at RPE 3–4
5	Rest	**Accelerations** 5:00 at RPE 2–3 5:00 at RPE 3–4 11:00 acceleration 10:00 at RPE 2–3 3:00 acceleration 10:00 at RPE 2–3	**Foundation Run** 5:00 at RPE 2–3 30:00 at RPE 3–4	**Foundation Run** 5:00 at RPE 2–3 30:00 at RPE 3–4

How to Run the Perfect Race

LEVEL

SSP   Steady-State Pace
LTP   Lactate Threshold Pace
CV   Critical Velocity
MAS   Maximal Aerobic Speed

5KP   5K Pace
10KP   10K Pace
HMP   Half-Marathon Pace

FRIDAY	SATURDAY	SUNDAY
Progression Run 5:00 at RPE 2–3 15:00 at RPE 3–4 8:00 at SSP 4:00 at LTP 2:00 at CV 5:00 at RPE 2–3	**Foundation Run** 5:00 at RPE 2–3 25:00 at RPE 3–4	**Endurance Run** 5:00 at RPE 2–3 30:00 at RPE 3–4 5:00 at RPE 4–5
Progression Run 5:00 at RPE 2–3 25:00 at RPE 3–4 4:00 at LTP 2:00 at CV 1:00 at MAS 5:00 at RPE 2–3	**Foundation Run** 5:00 at RPE 2–3 25:00 at RPE 3–4	**Endurance Run** 5:00 at RPE 2–3 40:00 at RPE 3–4 5:00 at RPE 4–5
Mini Intervals 5:00 at RPE 2–3 5:00 at RPE 3–4 30 × (0:30 at 10KP / 0:30 at RPE 2–3) 10:00 at RPE 2–3	**Foundation Run** 5:00 at RPE 2–3 25:00 at RPE 3–4	**Endurance Run** 5:00 at RPE 2–3 30:00 at RPE 3–4 5:00 at RPE 4–5
Tempo Run 5:00 at RPE 2–3 5:00 at RPE 3–4 12:00 at RPE 6 5:00 at RPE 2–3 12:00 at RPE 6 10:00 at RPE 2–3	**Foundation Run** 5:00 at RPE 2–3 30:00 at RPE 3–4	**Endurance Run** 5:00 at RPE 2–3 50:00 at RPE 3–4 5:00 at RPE 4–5
Critical Velocity Intervals 5:00 at RPE 2–3 5:00 at RPE 3–4 5 × 4:00 at RPE 6–7 / 2:00 at RPE 2–3 10:00 at RPE 2–3	**Foundation Run** 5:00 at RPE 2–3 30:00 at RPE 3–4	**Endurance Run** 5:00 at RPE 2–3 1:00:00 at RPE 3–4 5:00 at RPE 4–5

1   **10K**

	MONDAY	TUESDAY	WEDNESDAY	THURSDAY
6	Rest	**Hill Repetitions** 5:00 at RPE 2–3 5:00 at RPE 3–4 6 × 1:00 uphill at RPE 8–9 / 2:00 at RPE 2–3 10:00 at RPE 2–3	**Foundation Run** 5:00 at RPE 2–3 30:00 at RPE 3–4	**Foundation Run** 5:00 at RPE 2–3 30:00 at RPE 3–4
7	Rest	**5K Pace Intervals** 1 km at RPE 2–3 1 km at RPE 3–4 8 × (0.6 km at 5KP / 1:00 rest) 2 km at RPE 2–3	**Foundation Run** 5:00 at RPE 2–3 35:00 at RPE 3–4	**Foundation Run** 5:00 at RPE 2–3 35:00 at RPE 3–4
8	Rest	**Speed Intervals** 5:00 at RPE 2–3 5:00 at RPE 3–4 8 × 1:00 at RPE 8–9 / 2:00 at RPE 2–3 10:00 at RPE 2–3	**Foundation Run** 5:00 at RPE 2–3 35:00 at RPE 3–4	**Foundation Run** 5:00 at RPE 2–3 35:00 at RPE 3–4
9	Rest	**Accelerations** 5:00 at RPE 2–3 5:00 at RPE 3–4 11:00 acceleration 10:00 at RPE 2–3 6:00 acceleration 10:00 at RPE 2–3	**Foundation Run** 5:00 at RPE 2–3 30:00 at RPE 3–4	**Foundation Run** 5:00 at RPE 2–3 30:00 at RPE 3–4
10	Rest	**The Prefontaine** 1 km at RPE 2–3 1 km at RPE 3–4 ? × 200m at RPE 9 / 200m at RPE 6 1 km at RPE 2–3 1 km at RPE 3–4 *(? = Go to failure)*	**Foundation Run** 5:00 at RPE 2–3 40:00 at RPE 3–4	**Foundation Run** 5:00 at RPE 2–3 40:00 at RPE 3–4
11	Rest	**5K Pace Intervals** 1 km at RPE 2–3 1 km at RPE 3–4 6 × (0.8 km at 5KP / 1:00 rest) 2 km at RPE 2–3	**Foundation Run** 5:00 at RPE 2–3 40:00 at RPE 3–4	**Foundation Run** 5:00 at RPE 2–3 40:00 at RPE 3–4
12	Rest	**Fartleks** 5:00 at RPE 2–3 5:00 at RPE 3–4 8 × 1:00 at RPE 7–8 / 2:00 at RPE 2–3 10:00 at RPE 3–4	**Foundation Run** 5:00 at RPE 2–3 30:00 at RPE 3–4	**Fast Finish Run** 5:00 at RPE 2–3 25:00 at RPE 3–4 5:00 at RPE 6–7

FRIDAY	SATURDAY	SUNDAY
Progression Run 5:00 at RPE 2–3 20:00 at RPE 3–4 12:00 at SSP 6:00 at LTP 3:00 at CV 5:00 at RPE 2–3	**Foundation Run** 5:00 at RPE 2–3 30:00 at RPE 3–4	**Endurance Run** 5:00 at RPE 2–3 40:00 at RPE 3–4 5:00 at RPE 4–5
Steady-State Run 5:00 at RPE 2–3 5:00 at RPE 3–4 30:00 at RPE 5 10:00 at RPE 2–3	**Foundation Run** 5:00 at RPE 2–3 35:00 at RPE 3–4	**Endurance Run** 5:00 at RPE 2–3 1:10:00 at RPE 3–4 5:00 at RPE 4–5
Tempo Run 5:00 at RPE 2–3 5:00 at RPE 3–4 14:00 at RPE 6 5:00 at RPE 2–3 14:00 at RPE 6 10:00 at RPE 2–3	**Foundation Run** 5:00 at RPE 2–3 35:00 at RPE 3–4	**Endurance Run** 5:00 at RPE 2–3 1:10:00 at RPE 3–4 5:00 at RPE 4–5
Mini Intervals 5:00 at RPE 2–3 5:00 at RPE 3–4 30 × (0:30 at CV / 0:30 at RPE 2–3) 10:00 at RPE 2–3	**Foundation Run** 5:00 at RPE 2–3 30:00 at RPE 3–4	**Endurance Run** 5:00 at RPE 2–3 1:00:00 at RPE 3–4 5:00 at RPE 4–5
Critical Velocity Intervals 5:00 at RPE 2–3 5:00 at RPE 3–4 6 × 4:00 at RPE 6–7 / 2:00 at RPE 2–3 10:00 at RPE 2–3	**Foundation Run** 5:00 at RPE 2–3 40:00 at RPE 3–4	**Half-Marathon Pace Run** 1 km at RPE 2–3 1 km at RPE 3–4 3 × (3 km at HMP / 1:00 rest) 2 km at RPE 2–3
10K Pace Intervals 1 km at RPE 2–3 1 km at RPE 3–4 8 × (1 km at 10KP / 1:00 rest) 2 km at RPE 2–3	**Foundation Run** 5:00 at RPE 2–3 40:00 at RPE 3–4	**Endurance Run** 5:00 at RPE 2–3 1:00:00 at RPE 3–4 5:00 at RPE 4–5
Foundation Run 5:00 at RPE 2–3 15:00 at RPE 3–4	**10K Race**	Rest

1　10K

10K

This plan is a good fit for experienced competitive runners who are prepared to train hard in pursuit of improved 10K performance. Before starting the plan, be sure to build your training to the point where you're comfortably able to run 7 days a week for up to 70 minutes.

	MONDAY	TUESDAY	WEDNESDAY	THURSDAY
1	**Recovery Run** 30:00 at RPE 2–3	**Fartleks** 5:00 at RPE 2–3 10:00 at RPE 3–4 8 × 0:20 at RPE 8–9 / 1:40 at RPE 2–3 15:00 at RPE 3–4	**Foundation Run** 5:00 at RPE 2–3 40:00 at RPE 3–4	**Foundation Run** 5:00 at RPE 2–3 40:00 at RPE 3–4
2	**Recovery Run** 30:00 at RPE 2–3	**Fartleks** 5:00 at RPE 2–3 10:00 at RPE 3–4 8 × 1:00 at RPE 7–8 / 2:00 at RPE 2–3 15:00 at RPE 3–4	**Foundation Run** 5:00 at RPE 2–3 40:00 at RPE 3–4	**Foundation Run** 5:00 at RPE 2–3 40:00 at RPE 3–4
3	Rest	**Hill Repetitions** 5:00 at RPE 2–3 10:00 at RPE 3–4 8 × 0:30 uphill at RPE 8–9 / 1:30 at RPE 2–3 15:00 at RPE 2–3	**Foundation Run** 5:00 at RPE 2–3 40:00 at RPE 3–4	**Foundation Run** 5:00 at RPE 2–3 40:00 at RPE 3–4
4	**Recovery Run** 30:00 at RPE 2–3	**VO₂max Intervals** 5:00 at RPE 2–3 10:00 at RPE 3–4 6 × 2:00 at RPE 7–8 / 1:00 at RPE 2–3 15:00 at RPE 2–3	**Foundation Run** 5:00 at RPE 2–3 45:00 at RPE 3–4	**Foundation Run** 5:00 at RPE 2–3 45:00 at RPE 3–4
5	**Recovery Run** 30:00 at RPE 2–3	**Accelerations** 5:00 at RPE 2–3 10:00 at RPE 3–4 11:00 acceleration 10:00 at RPE 2–3 6:00 acceleration 15:00 at RPE 2–3	**Foundation Run** 5:00 at RPE 2–3 45:00 at RPE 3–4	**Foundation Run** 5:00 at RPE 2–3 45:00 at RPE 3–4

LEVEL

2

SSP   Steady-State Pace
LTP   Lactate Threshold Pace
CV   Critical Velocity
MAS   Maximal Aerobic Speed

5KP   5K Pace
10KP   10K Pace
HMP   Half-Marathon Pace

FRIDAY	SATURDAY	SUNDAY
Progression Run 5:00 at RPE 2–3 25:00 at RPE 3–4 8:00 at SSP 4:00 at LTP 2:00 at CV 5:00 at RPE 2–3	**Foundation Run** 5:00 at RPE 2–3 40:00 at RPE 3–4	**Endurance Run** 5:00 at RPE 2–3 1:00:00 at RPE 3–4 5:00 at RPE 4–5
Progression Run 5:00 at RPE 2–3 35:00 at RPE 3–4 4:00 at LTP 2:00 at CV 1:00 at MAS 5:00 at RPE 2–3	**Foundation Run** 5:00 at RPE 2–3 40:00 at RPE 3–4	**Endurance Run** 5:00 at RPE 2–3 1:10:00 at RPE 3–4 5:00 at RPE 4–5
Fartleks 5:00 at RPE 2–3 10:00 at RPE 3–4 1:00 at CV, 1:00 at RPE 2–3 2:00 at LTP, 1:00 at RPE 2–3 3:00 at SSP, 1:00 at RPE 2–3 2:00 at LTP, 1:00 at RPE 2–3 1:00 at CV, 1:00 at RPE 2–3 2:00 at LTP, 1:00 at RPE 2–3 3:00 at SSP, 1:00 at RPE 2–3 15:00 at RPE 3–4	**Foundation Run** 5:00 at RPE 2–3 40:00 at RPE 3–4	**Endurance Run** 5:00 at RPE 2–3 1:00:00 at RPE 3–4 5:00 at RPE 4–5
Critical Velocity Intervals 5:00 at RPE 2–3 10:00 at RPE 3–4 6 × 4:00 at RPE 6–7 / 2:00 at RPE 2–3 15:00 at RPE 2–3	**Foundation Run** 5:00 at RPE 2–3 45:00 at RPE 3–4	**Steady-State Run** 5:00 at RPE 2–3 10:00 at RPE 3–4 30:00 at RPE 5 15:00 at RPE 2–3
10K Pace Intervals 1 km at RPE 2–3 2 km at RPE 3–4 8 × (1 km at 10KP / 1:00 rest) 3 km at RPE 2–3	**Foundation Run** 5:00 at RPE 2–3 45:00 at RPE 3–4	**Mini Intervals** 10:00 at RPE 2–3 5:00 at RPE 3–4 40 × (0:30 at 10KP / 0:30 at RPE 2–3) 15:00 at RPE 2–3

	MONDAY	TUESDAY	WEDNESDAY	THURSDAY
6	Rest	**Speed Intervals** 5:00 at RPE 2–3 10:00 at RPE 3–4 8 × 1:00 at RPE 8–9 / 2:00 at RPE 2–3 15:00 at RPE 2–3	**Foundation Run** 5:00 at RPE 2–3 45:00 at RPE 3–4	**Foundation Run** 5:00 at RPE 2–3 45:00 at RPE 3–4
7	**Recovery Run** 30:00 at RPE 2–3	**5K Pace Intervals** 1 km at RPE 2–3 2 km at RPE 3–4 8 × (0.6 km at 5KP / 1:00 rest) 3 km at RPE 2–3	**Foundation Run** 5:00 at RPE 2–3 50:00 at RPE 3–4	**Foundation Run** 5:00 at RPE 2–3 50:00 at RPE 3–4
8	**Recovery Run** 30:00 at RPE 2–3	**Hill Repetitions** 5:00 at RPE 2–3 10:00 at RPE 3–4 10 × 1:00 uphill at RPE 8–9 / 2:00 at RPE 2–3 15:00 at RPE 2–3	**Foundation Run** 5:00 at RPE 2–3 50:00 at RPE 3–4	**Foundation Run** 5:00 at RPE 2–3 50:00 at RPE 3–4
9	Rest	**Accelerations** 5:00 at RPE 2–3 5:00 at RPE 3–4 11:00 acceleration 10:00 at RPE 2–3 6:00 acceleration 10:00 at RPE 2–3 3:00 acceleration 10:00 at RPE 2–3	**Foundation Run** 5:00 at RPE 2–3 50:00 at RPE 3–4	**Foundation Run** 5:00 at RPE 2–3 50:00 at RPE 3–4
10	**Recovery Run** 30:00 at RPE 2–3	**The Prefontaine** 1 km at RPE 2–3 2.5 km at RPE 3–4 ? × 200m at RPE 9 / 200m at RPE 6 1 km at RPE 2–3 2.5 km at RPE 3–4 *(? = Go to failure)*	**Foundation Run** 5:00 at RPE 2–3 55:00 at RPE 3–4	**Foundation Run** 5:00 at RPE 2–3 55:00 at RPE 3–4
11	**Recovery Run** 30:00 at RPE 2–3	**5K Pace Intervals** 1 km at RPE 2–3 2 km at RPE 3–4 6 × (0.8 km at 5KP / 1:00 rest) 3 km at RPE 2–3	**Foundation Run** 5:00 at RPE 2–3 55:00 at RPE 3–4	**Foundation Run** 5:00 at RPE 2–3 50:00 at RPE 3–4
12	Rest	**Fartleks** 5:00 at RPE 2–3 10:00 at RPE 3–4 8 × 1:00 at RPE 7–8 / 2:00 at RPE 2–3 15:00 at RPE 3–4	**Foundation Run** 5:00 at RPE 2–3 40:00 at RPE 3–4	**Fast Finish Run** 5:00 at RPE 2–3 25:00 at RPE 3–4 5:00 at RPE 6–7

FRIDAY	SATURDAY	SUNDAY
Progression Run 5:00 at RPE 2–3 20:00 at RPE 3–4 12:00 at SSP 6:00 at LTP 3:00 at CV 5:00 at RPE 2–3	**Foundation Run** 5:00 at RPE 2–3 45:00 at RPE 3–4	**Endurance Run** 5:00 at RPE 2–3 1:20:00 at RPE 3–4 5:00 at RPE 4–5
Half-Marathon Pace Run 1 km at RPE 2–3 2 km at RPE 3–4 3 × (3 km at HMP / 1:00 rest) 3 km at RPE 2–3	**Foundation Run** 5:00 at RPE 2–3 50:00 at RPE 3–4	**Tempo Run** 5:00 at RPE 2–3 10:00 at RPE 3–4 10:00 at RPE 6, 5:00 at RPE 2–3 10:00 at RPE 6, 5:00 at RPE 2–3 10:00 at RPE 6, 5:00 at RPE 2–3 15:00 at RPE 2–3
Critical Velocity Intervals 5:00 at RPE 2–3 10:00 at RPE 3–4 7 × 4:00 at RPE 6–7 / 2:00 at RPE 2–3 15:00 at RPE 2–3	**Foundation Run** 5:00 at RPE 2–3 50:00 at RPE 3–4	**Steady-State Run** 5:00 at RPE 2–3 10:00 at RPE 3–4 40:00 at RPE 5 15:00 at RPE 2–3
Fartleks 5:00 at RPE 2–3 10:00 at RPE 3–4 1:00 at CV, 1:00 at RPE 2–3 2:00 at LTP, 1:00 at RPE 2–3 3:00 at SSP, 1:00 at RPE 2–3 2:00 at LTP, 1:00 at RPE 2–3 1:00 at CV, 1:00 at RPE 2–3 2:00 at LTP, 1:00 at RPE 2–3 3:00 at SSP, 1:00 at RPE 2–3 15:00 at RPE 3–4	**Foundation Run** 5:00 at RPE 2–3 50:00 at RPE 3–4	**Endurance Run** 5:00 at RPE 2–3 1:30:00 at RPE 3–4 5:00 at RPE 4–5
10K Relaxed Time Trial 1 km at RPE 2–3 2 km at RPE 3–4 10 km at 95% effort 3 km at RPE 2–3	**Foundation Run** 5:00 at RPE 2–3 55:00 at RPE 3–4	**Mini Intervals** 5:00 at RPE 2–3 10:00 at RPE 3–4 40 × (0:30 at CV / 0:30 at RPE 2–3) 15:00 at RPE 2–3
10K Pace Intervals 1 km at RPE 2–3 2 km at RPE 3–4 10 × (1 km at 10KP / 1:00 rest) 3 km at RPE 2–3	**Foundation Run** 5:00 at RPE 2–3 45:00 at RPE 3–4	**Endurance Run** 5:00 at RPE 2–3 1:00:00 at RPE 3–4 5:00 at RPE 4–5
Foundation Run 5:00 at RPE 2–3 15:00 at RPE 3–4	**10K Race**	Rest

10K

This plan is designed for serious, competitive runners seeking the absolute limit of their potential at the 10K distance. Before starting the plan, be sure to build your training to the point where you're comfortably able to run nine times per week for up to 80 minutes.

	MONDAY	TUESDAY	WEDNESDAY	THURSDAY
1	**Recovery Run** 40:00 at RPE 2–3	**Fartleks** 5:00 at RPE 2–3 15:00 at RPE 3–4 10 × 0:20 at RPE 8–9 / 1:40 at RPE 2–3 20:00 at RPE 3–4 **Recovery Run** 20:00 at RPE 2–3	**Foundation Run** 5:00 at RPE 2–3 55:00 at RPE 3–4	**Foundation Run** 5:00 at RPE 2–3 55:00 at RPE 3–4
2	**Recovery Run** 40:00 at RPE 2–3	**Fartleks** 5:00 at RPE 2–3 15:00 at RPE 3–4 10 × 1:00 at RPE 7–8 / 2:00 at RPE 2–3 20:00 at RPE 3–4 **Recovery Run** 20:00 at RPE 2–3	**Foundation Run** 5:00 at RPE 2–3 55:00 at RPE 3–4	**Foundation Run** 5:00 at RPE 2–3 55:00 at RPE 3–4
3	Rest	**Hill Repetitions** 5:00 at RPE 2–3 15:00 at RPE 3–4 10 × 0:30 uphill at RPE 8–9 / 1:30 at RPE 2–3 20:00 at RPE 2–3 **Recovery Run** 20:00 at RPE 2–3	**Foundation Run** 5:00 at RPE 2–3 45:00 at RPE 3–4	**Foundation Run** 5:00 at RPE 2–3 50:00 at RPE 3–4

LEVEL

SSP Steady-State Pace
LTP Lactate Threshold Pace
CV Critical Velocity
MAS Maximal Aerobic Speed

5KP 5K Pace
10KP 10K Pace
HMP Half-Marathon Pace

FRIDAY	SATURDAY	SUNDAY
Progression Run 5:00 at RPE 2–3 35:00 at RPE 3–4 8:00 at SSP 4:00 at LTP 2:00 at CV 5:00 at RPE 2–3 **Recovery Run** 20:00 at RPE 2–3	**Foundation Run** 5:00 at RPE 2–3 55:00 at RPE 3–4	**Endurance Run** 5:00 at RPE 2–3 1:10:00 at RPE 3–4 5:00 at RPE 4–5
Progression Run 5:00 at RPE 2–3 35:00 at RPE 3–4 8:00 at LTP 4:00 at CV 2:00 at MAS 5:00 at RPE 2–3 **Recovery Run** 20:00 at RPE 2–3	**Foundation Run** 5:00 at RPE 2–3 55:00 at RPE 3–4	**Endurance Run** 5:00 at RPE 2–3 1:30:00 at RPE 3–4 5:00 at RPE 4–5
Fartleks 5:00 at RPE 2–3 15:00 at RPE 3–4 1:00 at CV, 1:00 at RPE 2–3 2:00 at LTP, 1:00 at RPE 2–3 3:00 at SSP, 1:00 at RPE 2–3 2:00 at LTP, 1:00 at RPE 2–3 1:00 at CV, 1:00 at RPE 2–3 2:00 at LTP, 1:00 at RPE 2–3 3:00 at SSP, 1:00 at RPE 2–3 2:00 at LTP, 1:00 at RPE 2–3 1:00 at CV, 1:00 at RPE 2–3 20:00 at RPE 3–4 **Recovery Run** 20:00 at RPE 2–3	**Foundation Run** 5:00 at RPE 2–3 45:00 at RPE 3–4	**Endurance Run** 5:00 at RPE 2–3 1:10:00 at RPE 3–4 5:00 at RPE 4–5

3 10K

	MONDAY	TUESDAY	WEDNESDAY	THURSDAY
4	**Recovery Run** 40:00 at RPE 2–3	**VO₂max Intervals** 5:00 at RPE 2–3 15:00 at RPE 3–4 7 × 2:00 at RPE 7–8 / 1:00 at RPE 2–3 20:00 at RPE 2–3 **Recovery Run** 25:00 at RPE 2–3	**Foundation Run** 5:00 at RPE 2–3 55:00 at RPE 3–4	**Foundation Run** 5:00 at RPE 2–3 1:00:00 at RPE 3–4
5	**Recovery Run** 40:00 at RPE 2–3	**Accelerations** 5:00 at RPE 2–3 15:00 at RPE 3–4 11:00 acceleration 10:00 at RPE 2–3 6:00 acceleration 3:00 acceleration 20:00 at RPE 2–3 **Recovery Run** 25:00 at RPE 2–3	**Foundation Run** 5:00 at RPE 2–3 55:00 at RPE 3–4	**Foundation Run** 5:00 at RPE 2–3 1:00:00 at RPE 3–4
6	Rest	**Speed Intervals** 5:00 at RPE 2–3 15:00 at RPE 3–4 8 × 0:45 at RPE 8–9 / 1:45 at RPE 2–3 20:00 at RPE 2–3 **Recovery Run** 20:00 at RPE 2–3	**Foundation Run** 5:00 at RPE 2–3 50:00 at RPE 3–4	**Foundation Run** 5:00 at RPE 2–3 55:00 at RPE 3–4
7	**Recovery Run** 40:00 at RPE 2–3	**5K Pace Intervals** 1 km at RPE 2–3 3 km at RPE 3–4 8 × (0.6 km at 5KP / 1:00 rest) 4 km at RPE 2–3 **Recovery Run** 30:00 at RPE 2–3	**Foundation Run** 5:00 at RPE 2–3 55:00 at RPE 3–4	**Foundation Run** 5:00 at RPE 2–3 1:05:00 at RPE 3–4
8	**Recovery Run** 40:00 at RPE 2–3	**Hill Repetitions** 5:00 at RPE 2–3 15:00 at RPE 3–4 12 × 1:00 uphill at RPE 8–9 / 2:00 at RPE 2–3 20:00 at RPE 2–3 **Recovery Run** 30:00 at RPE 2–3	**Foundation Run** 5:00 at RPE 2–3 55:00 at RPE 3–4	**Foundation Run** 5:00 at RPE 2–3 1:05:00 at RPE 3–4

FRIDAY	SATURDAY	SUNDAY
Critical Velocity Intervals 5:00 at RPE 2–3 15:00 at RPE 3–4 7 × 4:00 at RPE 6–7 / 2:00 at RPE 2–3 20:00 at RPE 2–3 **Recovery Run** 25:00 at RPE 2–3	**Foundation Run** 5:00 at RPE 2–3 55:00 at RPE 3–4	**Steady-State Run** 5:00 at RPE 2–3 15:00 at RPE 3–4 40:00 at RPE 5 20:00 at RPE 2–3
10K Pace Intervals 1 km at RPE 2–3 3 km at RPE 3–4 8 × (1 km at 10KP / 1:00 rest) 4 km at RPE 2–3 **Recovery Run** 25:00 at RPE 2–3	**Foundation Run** 5:00 at RPE 2–3 55:00 at RPE 3–4	**Mini Intervals** 5:00 at RPE 2–3 15:00 at RPE 3–4 50 × (0:30 at 10KP / 0:30 at RPE 2–3) 20:00 at RPE 2–3
Progression Run 5:00 at RPE 2–3 30:00 at RPE 3–4 12:00 at SSP 6:00 at LTP 3:00 at CV 5:00 at RPE 2–3 **Recovery Run** 20:00 at RPE 2–3	**Foundation Run** 5:00 at RPE 2–3 50:00 at RPE 3–4	**Endurance Run** 5:00 at RPE 2–3 1:30:00 at RPE 3–4 5:00 at RPE 4–5
Half-Marathon Pace Run 1 km at RPE 2–3 3 km at RPE 3–4 3 × (3 km at HMP / 1:00 rest) 4 km at RPE 2–3 **Recovery Run** 30:00 at RPE 2–3	**Foundation Run** 5:00 at RPE 2–3 55:00 at RPE 3–4	**Tempo Run** 5:00 at RPE 2–3 15:00 at RPE 3–4 10:00 at RPE 6, 5:00 at RPE 2–3 10:00 at RPE 6, 5:00 at RPE 2–3 10:00 at RPE 6, 5:00 at RPE 2–3 20:00 at RPE 2–3
Critical Velocity Intervals 5:00 at RPE 2–3 15:00 at RPE 3–4 8 × 4:00 at RPE 6–7 / 2:00 at RPE 2–3 15:00 at RPE 2–3 **Recovery Run** 30:00 at RPE 2–3	**Foundation Run** 5:00 at RPE 2–3 55:00 at RPE 3–4	**Steady-State Run** 5:00 at RPE 2–3 15:00 at RPE 3–4 50:00 at RPE 5 20:00 at RPE 2–3

3 **10K**

	MONDAY	TUESDAY	WEDNESDAY	THURSDAY
9	Rest	**Accelerations** 5:00 at RPE 2–3 15:00 at RPE 3–4 11:00 acceleration 10:00 at RPE 2–3 6:00 acceleration 3:00 acceleration 20:00 at RPE 2–3 **Recovery Run** 25:00 at RPE 2–3	**Foundation Run** 5:00 at RPE 2–3 55:00 at RPE 3–4	**Foundation Run** 5:00 at RPE 2–3 55:00 at RPE 3–4
10	**Recovery Run** 40:00 at RPE 2–3	**The Prefontaine** 1 km at RPE 2–3 4 km at RPE 3–4 ? × 200m at RPE 9 / 200m at RPE 6 1 km at RPE 2–3 4 km at RPE 3–4 *(? = Go to failure)* **Recovery Run** 35:00 at RPE 2–3	**Foundation Run** 5:00 at RPE 2–3 55:00 at RPE 3–4	**Foundation Run** 5:00 at RPE 2–3 1:10:00 at RPE 3–4
11	**Recovery Run** 40:00 at RPE 2–3	**5K Pace Intervals** 1 km at RPE 2–3 3 km at RPE 3–4 6 × (0.8 km at 5KP / 1:00 rest) 4 km at RPE 2–3 **Recovery Run** 30:00 at RPE 2–3	**Foundation Run** 5:00 at RPE 2–3 55:00 at RPE 3–4	**Foundation Run** 5:00 at RPE 2–3 55:00 at RPE 3–4
12	Rest	**Fartleks** 5:00 at RPE 2–3 15:00 at RPE 3–4 10 × 1:00 at RPE 7–8 / 2:00 at RPE 2–3 20:00 at RPE 3–4	**Foundation Run** 5:00 at RPE 2–3 40:00 at RPE 3–4	**Fast Finish Run** 5:00 at RPE 2–3 30:00 at RPE 3–4 5:00 at RPE 6–7

How to Run the Perfect Race

FRIDAY	SATURDAY	SUNDAY
Fartleks 5:00 at RPE 2–3 15:00 at RPE 3–4 1:00 at CV, 1:00 at RPE 2–3 2:00 at LTP, 1:00 at RPE 2–3 3:00 at SSP, 1:00 at RPE 2–3 2:00 at LTP, 1:00 at RPE 2–3 1:00 at CV, 1:00 at RPE 2–3 2:00 at LTP, 1:00 at RPE 2–3 3:00 at SSP, 1:00 at RPE 2–3 20:00 at RPE 3–4 **Recovery Run** 25:00 at RPE 2–3	**Foundation Run** 5:00 at RPE 2–3 55:00 at RPE 3–4	**Endurance Run** 5:00 at RPE 2–3 1:30:00 at RPE 3–4 5:00 at RPE 4–5
10K Relaxed Time Trial 1 km at RPE 2–3 3 km at RPE 3–4 10 km at 95% effort 4 km at RPE 2–3 **Recovery Run** 35:00 at RPE 2–3	**Foundation Run** 5:00 at RPE 2–3 55:00 at RPE 3–4	**Mini Intervals** 5:00 at RPE 2–3 15:00 at RPE 3–4 50 × (0:30 at CV / 0:30 at RPE 2–3) 20:00 at RPE 2–3
10K Pace Intervals 1 km at RPE 2–3 3 km at RPE 3–4 10 × (1 km at 10KP / 1:00 rest) 4 km at RPE 2–3 **Recovery Run** 30:00 at RPE 2–3	**Foundation Run** 5:00 at RPE 2–3 55:00 at RPE 3–4	**Endurance Run** 5:00 at RPE 2–3 1:00:00 at RPE 3–4 5:00 at RPE 4–5
Foundation Run 5:00 at RPE 2–3 15:00 at RPE 3–4	**10K Race**	Rest

3 10K

11

Half-Marathon Training Plans

The four training plans presented in this chapter are designed to help runners master the art of pacing and find their limit at the half-marathon distance. The various levels cover the needs of everyone from first-timers to elites. Refer back to Chapter 6 for details on the RPE-based intensity scale used throughout the plans and for full explanations of certain terms and workout types. Online versions of the plans are available for separate purchase on the 80/20 Endurance web site. Additionally, device-compatible free versions of the individual workouts can be found at https://www.8020endurance.com.

Half-Marathon

This plan is appropriate for beginning runners preparing for their first half-marathon event and for more experienced runners who need or prefer a relatively low-volume training program for any reason. Before starting the plan, be sure to build your training to the point where you're comfortably able to run 5 days a week for up to 40 minutes.

	MONDAY	TUESDAY	WEDNESDAY	THURSDAY
1	Rest	**Progression Run** 5:00 at RPE 2–3 10:00 at RPE 3–4 8:00 at SSP 4:00 at LTP 2:00 at CV 5:00 at RPE 2–3	**Foundation Run** 5:00 at RPE 2–3 25:00 at RPE 3–4	Rest
2	Rest	**Progression Run** 5:00 at RPE 2–3 20:00 at RPE 3–4 4:00 at LTP 2:00 at CV 1:00 at MAS 5:00 at RPE 2–3	**Foundation Run** 5:00 at RPE 2–3 30:00 at RPE 3–4	Rest
3	Rest	**Fartleks** 5:00 at RPE 2–3 5:00 at RPE 3–4 1:00 at CV, 1:00 at RPE 2–3 2:00 at LTP, 1:00 at RPE 2–3 3:00 at SSP, 1:00 at RPE 2–3 2:00 at LTP, 1:00 at RPE 2–3 1:00 at CV, 1:00 at RPE 2–3 10:00 at RPE 3–4	**Foundation Run** 5:00 at RPE 2–3 25:00 at RPE 3–4	Rest
4	Rest	**Critical Velocity Intervals** 5:00 at RPE 2–3 5:00 at RPE 3–4 4 × 4:00 at RPE 6–7* / 2:00 at RPE 2–3 10:00 at RPE 2–3 *Precision Splitting*	**Foundation Run** 5:00 at RPE 2–3 30:00 at RPE 3–4	Rest
5	Rest	**Mini Intervals** 5:00 at RPE 2–3 5:00 at RPE 3–4 20 × (0:30 at 10KP / 0:30 at RPE 2–3) 10:00 at RPE 2–3	**Foundation Run** 5:00 at RPE 2–3 35:00 at RPE 3–4	Rest

LEVEL

SSP Steady-State Pace
LTP Lactate Threshold Pace
CV Critical Velocity
MAS Maximal Aerobic Speed

5KP 5K Pace
10KP 10K Pace

FRIDAY	SATURDAY	SUNDAY
Fartleks 5:00 at RPE 2–3 5:00 at RPE 3–4 6 × 0:20 at RPE 8–9 / 1:40 at RPE 2–3 10:00 at RPE 3–4	**Foundation Run** 5:00 at RPE 2–3 25:00 at RPE 3–4	**Endurance Run** 5:00 at RPE 2–3 30:00 at RPE 3–4 5:00 at RPE 4–5
Fartleks 5:00 at RPE 2–3 5:00 at RPE 3–4 6 × 1:00 at RPE 7–8 / 2:00 at RPE 2–3 10:00 at RPE 3–4	**Foundation Run** 5:00 at RPE 2–3 30:00 at RPE 3–4	**Endurance Run** 5:00 at RPE 2–3 40:00 at RPE 3–4 5:00 at RPE 4–5
Hill Repetitions 5:00 at RPE 2–3 5:00 at RPE 3–4 6 × 0:30 uphill at RPE 8–9* / 1:30 at RPE 2–3 10:00 at RPE 2–3 *Stretch Intervals*	**Foundation Run** 5:00 at RPE 2–3 25:00 at RPE 3–4	**Endurance Run** 5:00 at RPE 2–3 35:00 at RPE 3–4 5:00 at RPE 4–5
VO$_2$max Intervals 5:00 at RPE 2–3 5:00 at RPE 3–4 4 × 2:00 at RPE 7–8* / 2:00 at RPE 2–3 10:00 at RPE 2–3 *Precision Splitting*	**Foundation Run** 5:00 at RPE 2–3 30:00 at RPE 3–4	**Endurance Run** 5:00 at RPE 2–3 50:00 at RPE 3–4 5:00 at RPE 4–5
Accelerations 5:00 at RPE 2–3 5:00 at RPE 3–4 11:00 acceleration 10:00 at RPE 2–3 3:00 acceleration 10:00 at RPE 2–3	**Foundation Run** 5:00 at RPE 2–3 35:00 at RPE 3–4	**Endurance Run** 5:00 at RPE 2–3 1:00:00 at RPE 3–4 5:00 at RPE 4–5

	MONDAY	TUESDAY	WEDNESDAY	THURSDAY
6	Rest	**Progression Run** 5:00 at RPE 2–3 15:00 at RPE 3–4 12:00 at SSP 8:00 at LTP 4:00 at CV 5:00 at RPE 2–3	**Foundation Run** 5:00 at RPE 2–3 30:00 at RPE 3–4	Rest
7	Rest	**Tempo Run** 5:00 at RPE 2–3 5:00 at RPE 3–4 12:00 at RPE 6 5:00 at RPE 2–3 12:00 at RPE 6 10:00 at RPE 2–3	**Foundation Run** 5:00 at RPE 2–3 35:00 at RPE 3–4	Rest
8	Rest	**Steady-State Run** 5:00 at RPE 2–3 5:00 at RPE 3–4 30:00 at RPE 5 10:00 at RPE 2–3	**Foundation Run** 5:00 at RPE 2–3 40:00 at RPE 3–4	Rest
9	Rest	**Fartleks** 5:00 at RPE 2–3 5:00 at RPE 3–4 1:00 at CV, 1:00 at RPE 2–3 2:00 at LTP, 1:00 at RPE 2–3 3:00 at SSP, 1:00 at RPE 2–3 2:00 at LTP, 1:00 at RPE 2–3 1:00 at CV, 1:00 at RPE 2–3 2:00 at LTP, 1:00 at RPE 2–3 1:00 at CV, 1:00 at RPE 2–3 10:00 at RPE 3–4	**Foundation Run** 5:00 at RPE 2–3 35:00 at RPE 3–4	Rest
10	Rest	**Critical Velocity Intervals** 5:00 at RPE 2–3 5:00 at RPE 3–4 5 × 4:00 at RPE 6–7* / 2:00 at RPE 2–3 10:00 at RPE 2–3 *Precision Splitting*	**Foundation Run** 5:00 at RPE 2–3 40:00 at RPE 3–4	Rest
11	Rest	**Mini Intervals** 5:00 at RPE 2–3 5:00 at RPE 3–4 20 × (0:30 at CV / 0:30 at RPE 2–3) 10:00 at RPE 2–3	**Foundation Run** 5:00 at RPE 2–3 40:00 at RPE 3–4	Rest

How to Run the Perfect Race

FRIDAY	SATURDAY	SUNDAY
Speed Intervals 5;00 at RPE 2–3 5:00 at RPE 3–4 6 × 0:45 at RPE 8–9* / 1:45 at RPE 2–3 10:00 at RPE 2–3 *Stretch Intervals*	**Foundation Run** 5:00 at RPE 2–3 30:00 at RPE 3–4	**Endurance Run** 5:00 at RPE 2–3 50:00 at RPE 3–4 5:00 at RPE 4–5
5K Pace Intervals 1 km at RPE 2–3 1 km at RPE 3–4 8 × (0.6 km at 5KP* / 1:00 rest) 2 km at RPE 2–3 *Precision Splitting*	**Foundation Run** 5:00 at RPE 2–3 35:00 at RPE 3–4	**Endurance Run** 5:00 at RPE 2–3 1:10:00 at RPE 3–4 5:00 at RPE 4–5
VO₂max Intervals 5:00 at RPE 2–3 5:00 at RPE 3–4 5 × 2:00 at RPE 7–8* / 2:00 at RPE 2–3 10:00 at RPE 2–3 *Precision Splitting*	**Foundation Run** 5:00 at RPE 2–3 40:00 at RPE 3–4	**Endurance Run** 5:00 at RPE 2–3 1:20:00 at RPE 3–4 5:00 at RPE 4–5
Hill Repetitions 5:00 at RPE 2–3 5:00 at RPE 3–4 6 × 1:00 uphill at RPE 8–9* / 2:00 at RPE 2–3 10:00 at RPE 2–3 *Stretch Intervals*	**Foundation Run** 5:00 at RPE 2–3 35:00 at RPE 3–4	**Endurance Run** 5:00 at RPE 2–3 1:00:00 at RPE 3–4 5:00 at RPE 4–5
5K Pace Intervals 1 km at RPE 2–3 1 km at RPE 3–4 6 × (0.8 km at 5KP* / 1:00 rest) 2 km at RPE 2–3 *Precision Splitting*	**Foundation Run** 5:00 at RPE 2–3 40:00 at RPE 3–4	**Endurance Run** 5:00 at RPE 2–3 1:30:00 at RPE 3–4 5:00 at RPE 4–5
Accelerations 5:00 at RPE 2–3 5:00 at RPE 3–4 11:00 acceleration 10:00 at RPE 2–3 6:00 acceleration 10:00 at RPE 2–3	**Foundation Run** 5:00 at RPE 2–3 40:00 at RPE 3–4	**Endurance Run** 5:00 at RPE 2–3 1:40:00 at RPE 3–4 5:00 at RPE 4–5

Half-Marathon

	MONDAY	TUESDAY	WEDNESDAY	THURSDAY
12	Rest	**Progression Run** 5:00 at RPE 2–3 30:00 at RPE 3–4 8:00 at LTP 4:00 at CV 2:00 at MAS 5:00 at RPE 2–3	**Foundation Run** 5:00 at RPE 2–3 35:00 at RPE 3–4	Rest
13	Rest	**Tempo Run** 5:00 at RPE 2–3 5:00 at RPE 3–4 14:00 at RPE 6 5:00 at RPE 2–3 14:00 at RPE 6 10:00 at RPE 2–3	**Foundation Run** 5:00 at RPE 2–3 40:00 at RPE 3–4	Rest
14	Rest	**Steady-State Run** 5:00 at RPE 2–3 5:00 at RPE 3–4 40:00 at RPE 5 10:00 at RPE 2–3	**Foundation Run** 5:00 at RPE 2–3 40:00 at RPE 3–4	Rest
15	Rest	**Fartleks** 5:00 at RPE 2–3 5:00 at RPE 3–4 6 × 1:00 at RPE 7–8 / 2:00 at RPE 2–3 10:00 at RPE 3–4	**Foundation Run** 5:00 at RPE 2–3 40:00 at RPE 3–4	Rest

How to Run the Perfect Race

FRIDAY	SATURDAY	SUNDAY
Speed Intervals 5:00 at RPE 2–3 5:00 at RPE 3–4 8 × 0:45 at RPE 8–9* / 1:45 at RPE 2–3 10:00 at RPE 2–3 *Stretch Intervals*	**Foundation Run** 5:00 at RPE 2–3 35:00 at RPE 3–4	**Endurance Run** 5:00 at RPE 2–3 1.10.00 at RPE 3–4 5:00 at RPE 4–5
VO₂max Intervals 5:00 at RPE 2–3 5:00 at RPE 3–4 5 × 2:00 at RPE 7–8* / 2:00 at RPE 2–3 10:00 at RPE 2–3 *Precision Splitting*	**Foundation Run** 5:00 at RPE 2–3 40:00 at RPE 3–4	**Endurance Run** 5:00 at RPE 2–3 1:50:00 at RPE 3–4 5:00 at RPE 4–5
Relaxed 5K Time Trial 1 km at RPE 2–3 1 km at RPE 3–4 5 km at 95% effort 2 km at RPE 2–3	**Foundation Run** 5:00 at RPE 2–3 40:00 at RPE 3–4	**Endurance Run** 5:00 at RPE 2–3 1:10:00 at RPE 3–4 5:00 at RPE 4–5
Fast Finish Run 5:00 at RPE 2–3 10:00 at RPE 3–4 5:00 at RPE 6–7	**Foundation Run** 5:00 at RPE 2–3 15:00 at RPE 3–4	**Half-Marathon Race**

Half-Marathon

Half-Marathon

This plan is designed for runners who are ready to take their training load up a notch in order to improve their half-marathon time. Before starting the plan, be sure to build your training to the point where you're comfortably able to run 6 days a week for up to 1 hour.

	MONDAY	TUESDAY	WEDNESDAY	THURSDAY
1	Rest	**Progression Run** 5:00 at RPE 2–3 10:00 at RPE 3–4 8:00 at SSP 4:00 at LTP 2:00 at CV 5:00 at RPE 2–3	**Foundation Run** 5:00 at RPE 2–3 25:00 at RPE 3–4	**Foundation Run** 5:00 at RPE 2–3 25:00 at RPE 3–4
2	Rest	**Progression Run** 5:00 at RPE 2–3 25:00 at RPE 3–4 4:00 at LTP 2:00 at CV 1:00 at MAS 5:00 at RPE 2–3	**Foundation Run** 5:00 at RPE 2–3 30:00 at RPE 3–4	**Foundation Run** 5:00 at RPE 2–3 30:00 at RPE 3–4
3	Rest	**Fartleks** 5:00 at RPE 2–3 5:00 at RPE 3–4 1:00 at CV, 1:00 at RPE 2–3 2:00 at LTP, 1:00 at RPE 2–3 3:00 at SSP, 1:00 at RPE 2–3 2:00 at LTP, 1:00 at RPE 2–3 1:00 at CV, 1:00 at RPE 2–3 2:00 at LTP, 1:00 at RPE 2–3 3:00 at SSP, 1:00 at RPE 2–3 10:00 at RPE 3–4	**Foundation Run** 5:00 at RPE 2–3 25:00 at RPE 3–4	**Foundation Run** 5:00 at RPE 2–3 25:00 at RPE 3–4
4	Rest	**Critical Velocity Intervals** 5:00 at RPE 2–3 5:00 at RPE 3–4 5 × 4:00 at RPE 6–7* / 2:00 at RPE 2–3 10:00 at RPE 2–3 *Precision Splitting*	**Foundation Run** 5:00 at RPE 2–3 30:00 at RPE 3–4	**Foundation Run** 5:00 at RPE 2–3 30:00 at RPE 3–4

SSP Steady-State Pace
LTP Lactate Threshold Pace
CV Critical Velocity
MAS Maximal Aerobic Speed

5KP 5K Pace
10KP 10K Pace
HMP Half-Marathon Pace

FRIDAY	SATURDAY	SUNDAY
Fartleks 5:00 at RPE 2–3 5:00 at RPE 3–4 6 × 0:20 at RPE 8–9 / 1:40 at RPE 2–3 10:00 at RPE 3–4	**Foundation Run** 5:00 at RPE 2–3 25:00 at RPE 3–4	**Endurance Run** 5:00 at RPE 2–3 50:00 at RPE 3–4 5:00 at RPE 4–5
Fartleks 5:00 at RPE 2–3 5:00 at RPE 3–4 6 × 1:00 at RPE 7–8 / 2:00 at RPE 2–3 10:00 at RPE 3–4	**Foundation Run** 5:00 at RPE 2–3 30:00 at RPE 3–4	**Endurance Run** 5:00 at RPE 2–3 1:00:00 at RPE 3–4 5:00 at RPE 4–5
Hill Repetitions 5:00 at RPE 2–3 5:00 at RPE 3–4 8 × 0:30 uphill at RPE 8–9* / 1:30 at RPE 2–3 10:00 at RPE 2–3 *Stretch Intervals	**Foundation Run** 5:00 at RPE 2–3 25:00 at RPE 3–4	**Endurance Run** 5:00 at RPE 2–3 50:00 at RPE 3–4 5:00 at RPE 4–5
VO$_2$max Intervals 5:00 at RPE 2–3 5:00 at RPE 3–4 5 × 2:00 at RPE 7–8* / 2:00 at RPE 2–3 10:00 at RPE 2–3 *Precision Splitting	**Foundation Run** 5:00 at RPE 2–3 30:00 at RPE 3–4	**Endurance Run** 5:00 at RPE 2–3 1:10:00 at RPE 3–4 5:00 at RPE 4–5

	MONDAY	TUESDAY	WEDNESDAY	THURSDAY
5	Rest	**Mini Intervals** 5:00 at RPE 2–3 5:00 at RPE 3–4 30 × (0:30 at 10KP / 0:30 at RPE 2–3) 10:00 at RPE 2–3	**Foundation Run** 5:00 at RPE 2–3 35:00 at RPE 3–4	**Foundation Run** 5:00 at RPE 2–3 35:00 at RPE 3–4
6	Rest	**Progression Run** 5:00 at RPE 2–3 20:00 at RPE 3–4 12:00 at SSP 8:00 at LTP 4:00 at CV 5:00 at RPE 2–3	**Foundation Run** 5:00 at RPE 2–3 30:00 at RPE 3–4	**Foundation Run** 5:00 at RPE 2–3 30:00 at RPE 3–4
7	Rest	**Tempo Run** 5:00 at RPE 2–3 5:00 at RPE 3–4 14:00 at RPE 6 5:00 at RPE 2–3 14:00 at RPE 6 10:00 at RPE 2–3	**Foundation Run** 5:00 at RPE 2–3 35:00 at RPE 3–4	**Foundation Run** 5:00 at RPE 2–3 35:00 at RPE 3–4
8	Rest	**Steady-State Run** 5:00 at RPE 2–3 5:00 at RPE 3–4 35:00 at RPE 5 10:00 at RPE 2–3	**Foundation Run** 5:00 at RPE 2–3 40:00 at RPE 3–4	**Foundation Run** 5:00 at RPE 2–3 40:00 at RPE 3–4
9	Rest	**Fartleks** 5:00 at RPE 2–3 5:00 at RPE 3–4 1:00 at CV, 1:00 at RPE 2–3 2:00 at LTP, 1:00 at RPE 2–3 3:00 at SSP, 1:00 at RPE 2–3 2:00 at LTP, 1:00 at RPE 2–3 1:00 at CV, 1:00 at RPE 2–3 2:00 at LTP, 1:00 at RPE 2–3 1:00 at CV, 1:00 at RPE 2–3 10:00 at RPE 3–4	**Foundation Run** 5:00 at RPE 2–3 35:00 at RPE 3–4	**Foundation Run** 5:00 at RPE 2–3 35:00 at RPE 3–4
10	Rest	**Critical Velocity Intervals** 5:00 at RPE 2–3 5:00 at RPE 3–4 6 × 4:00 at RPE 6–7* / 2:00 at RPE 2–3 10:00 at RPE 2–3 *Precision Splitting*	**Foundation Run** 5:00 at RPE 2–3 40:00 at RPE 3–4	**Foundation Run** 5:00 at RPE 2–3 40:00 at RPE 3–4

FRIDAY	SATURDAY	SUNDAY
Accelerations 5:00 at RPE 2–3 5:00 at RPE 3–4 11:00 acceleration 10:00 at RPE 2–3 6:00 acceleration 10:00 at RPE 2–3	**Foundation Run** 5:00 at RPE 2–3 35:00 at RPE 3–4	**Endurance Run** 5:00 at RPE 2–3 1:20:00 at RPE 3–4 5:00 at RPE 4–5
Speed Intervals 5:00 at RPE 2–3 5:00 at RPE 3–4 8 × 0:45 at RPE 8–9* / 1:45 at RPE 2–3 10:00 at RPE 2–3 *Stretch Intervals*	**Foundation Run** 5:00 at RPE 2–3 30:00 at RPE 3–4	**Endurance Run** 5:00 at RPE 2–3 1:00:00 at RPE 3–4 5:00 at RPE 4–5
5K Pace Intervals 1 km at RPE 2–3 1 km at RPE 3–4 6 × (0.8 km at 5KP* / 1:00 rest) 2 km at RPE 2–3 *Precision Splitting*	**Foundation Run** 5:00 at RPE 2–3 35:00 at RPE 3–4	**Endurance Run** 5:00 at RPE 2–3 1:30:00 at RPE 3–4 5:00 at RPE 4–5
VO₂max Intervals 5:00 at RPE 2–3 5:00 at RPE 3–4 6 × 2:00 at RPE 7–8* / 2:00 at RPE 2–3 10:00 at RPE 2–3 *Precision Splitting*	**Foundation Run** 5:00 at RPE 2–3 40:00 at RPE 3–4	**Half-Marathon Pace Run** 1 km at RPE 2–3 1 km at RPE 3–4 3 × (3 km at HMP / 1:00 rest) 2 km at RPE 2–3
Hill Repetitions 5:00 at RPE 2–3 5:00 at RPE 3–4 8 × 1:00 uphill at RPE 8–9* / 2:00 at RPE 2–3 10:00 at RPE 2–3 *Stretch Intervals*	**Foundation Run** 5:00 at RPE 2–3 35:00 at RPE 3–4	**Endurance Run** 5:00 at RPE 2–3 1:10:00 at RPE 3–4 5:00 at RPE 4–5
The Prefontaine 1 km at RPE 2–3 1 km at RPE 3–4 ? × 200m at RPE 9 / 200m at RPE 6 1 km at RPE 2–3 1 km at RPE 3–4 *(? = Go to failure)*	**Foundation Run** 5:00 at RPE 2–3 40:00 at RPE 3–4	**Endurance Run** 5:00 at RPE 2–3 1:40:00 at RPE 3–4 5:00 at RPE 4–5

1 Half-Marathon

	MONDAY	TUESDAY	WEDNESDAY	THURSDAY
11	Rest	**Mini Intervals** 5:00 at RPE 2–3 5:00 at RPE 3–4 30 × (0:30 at CV / 0:30 at RPE 2–3) 10:00 at RPE 2–3	**Foundation Run** 5:00 at RPE 2–3 45:00 at RPE 3–4	**Foundation Run** 5:00 at RPE 2–3 45:00 at RPE 3–4
12	Rest	**Progression Run** 5:00 at RPE 2–3 30:00 at RPE 3–4 8:00 at LTP 4:00 at CV 2:00 at MAS 5:00 at RPE 2–3	**Foundation Run** 5:00 at RPE 2–3 40:00 at RPE 3–4	**Foundation Run** 5:00 at RPE 2–3 40:00 at RPE 3–4
13	Rest	**Tempo Run** 5:00 at RPE 2–3 5:00 at RPE 3–4 16:00 at RPE 6 5:00 at RPE 2–3 16:00 at RPE 6 10:00 at RPE 2–3	**Foundation Run** 5:00 at RPE 2–3 45:00 at RPE 3–4	**Foundation Run** 5:00 at RPE 2–3 45:00 at RPE 3–4
14	Rest	**Steady-State Run** 5:00 at RPE 2–3 5:00 at RPE 3–4 45:00 at RPE 5 10:00 at RPE 2–3	**Foundation Run** 5:00 at RPE 2–3 40:00 at RPE 3–4	**Foundation Run** 5:00 at RPE 2–3 40:00 at RPE 3–4
15	Rest	**Fartleks** 5:00 at RPE 2–3 5:00 at RPE 3–4 8 × 1:00 at RPE 7–8 / 2:00 at RPE 2–3 10:00 at RPE 3–4	**Foundation Run** 5:00 at RPE 2–3 35:00 at RPE 3–4	**Foundation Run** 5:00 at RPE 2–3 25:00 at RPE 3–4

How to Run the Perfect Race

FRIDAY	SATURDAY	SUNDAY
Speed Intervals 5:00 at RPE 2–3 5:00 at RPE 3–4 8 × 0:45 at RPE 8–9* / 1:45 at RPE 2–3 10:00 at RPE 2–3 *Stretch Intervals*	**Foundation Run** 5:00 at RPE 2–3 45:00 at RPE 3–4	**Endurance Run** 5:00 at RPE 2–3 1:50:00 at RPE 3–4 5:00 at RPE 4–5
Accelerations 5:00 at RPE 2–3 5:00 at RPE 3–4 11:00 acceleration 10:00 at RPE 2–3 6:00 acceleration 10:00 at RPE 2–3	**Foundation Run** 5:00 at RPE 2–3 40:00 at RPE 3–4	**Endurance Run** 5:00 at RPE 2–3 1:10:00 at RPE 3–4 5:00 at RPE 4–5
VO₂max Intervals 5:00 at RPE 2–3 5:00 at RPE 3–4 6 × 2:00 at RPE 7–8* / 2:00 at RPE 2–3 10:00 at RPE 2–3 *Precision Splitting*	**Foundation Run** 5:00 at RPE 2–3 45:00 at RPE 3–4	**Half-Marathon Pace Run** 1 km at RPE 2–3 1 km at RPE 3–4 2 × (5 km at HMP / 1:00 rest) 2 km at RPE 2–3
Relaxed 5K Time Trial 1 km at RPE 2–3 1 km at RPE 3–4 5 km at 95% effort 2 km at RPE 2–3	**Foundation Run** 5:00 at RPE 2–3 40:00 at RPE 3–4	**Endurance Run** 5:00 at RPE 2–3 1:10:00 at RPE 3–4 5:00 at RPE 4–5
Fast Finish Run 5:00 at RPE 2–3 15:00 at RPE 3–4 5:00 at RPE 6–7	**Foundation Run** 5:00 at RPE 2–3 15:00 at RPE 3–4	**Half-Marathon Race**

Half-Marathon

1

Half-Marathon

This plan is a good fit for experienced competitive runners who are prepared to train hard in pursuit of improved half-marathon performance. Before starting the plan, be sure to build your training to the point where you're comfortably able to run 7 days a week for up to 80 minutes.

	MONDAY	TUESDAY	WEDNESDAY	THURSDAY
1	**Recovery Run** 30:00 at RPE 2–3	**Progression Run** 5:00 at RPE 2–3 25:00 at RPE 3–4 8:00 at SSP 4:00 at LTP 2:00 at CV 5:00 at RPE 2–3	**Foundation Run** 5:00 at RPE 2–3 40:00 at RPE 3–4	**Foundation Run** 5:00 at RPE 2–3 40:00 at RPE 3–4
2	**Recovery Run** 30:00 at RPE 2–3	**Progression Run** 5:00 at RPE 2–3 35:00 at RPE 3–4 4:00 at LTP 2:00 at CV 1:00 at MAS 5:00 at RPE 2–3	**Foundation Run** 5:00 at RPE 2–3 45:00 at RPE 3–4	**Foundation Run** 5:00 at RPE 2–3 45:00 at RPE 3–4
3	Rest	**Fartleks** 5:00 at RPE 2–3 10:00 at RPE 3–4 1:00 at CV, 1:00 at RPE 2–3 2:00 at LTP, 1:00 at RPE 2–3 3:00 at SSP, 1:00 at RPE 2–3 2:00 at LTP, 1:00 at RPE 2–3 1:00 at CV, 1:00 at RPE 2–3 2:00 at LTP, 1:00 at RPE 2–3 3:00 at SSP, 1:00 at RPE 2–3 15:00 at RPE 3–4	**Foundation Run** 5:00 at RPE 2–3 40:00 at RPE 3–4	**Foundation Run** 5:00 at RPE 2–3 40:00 at RPE 3–4
4	**Recovery Run** 30:00 at RPE 2–3	**Critical Velocity Intervals** 5:00 at RPE 2–3 10:00 at RPE 3–4 6 × 4:00* at RPE 6–7 / 2:00 at RPE 2–3 15:00 at RPE 2–3 *Precision Splitting*	**Foundation Run** 5:00 at RPE 2–3 45:00 at RPE 3–4	**Foundation Run** 5:00 at RPE 2–3 45:00 at RPE 3–4

How to Run the Perfect Race

SSP Steady-State Pace
LTP Lactate Threshold Pace
CV Critical Velocity
MAS Maximal Aerobic Speed

5KP 5K Pace
10KP 10K Pace
HMP Half-Marathon Pace

Half-Marathon

2

FRIDAY	SATURDAY	SUNDAY
Fartleks 5:00 at RPE 2–3 10:00 at RPE 3–4 8 × 0:20 at RPE 8–9 / 1:40 at RPE 2–3 15:00 at RPE 3–4	**Foundation Run** 5:00 at RPE 2–3 40:00 at RPE 3–4	**Endurance Run** 5:00 at RPE 2–3 1:10:00 at RPE 3–4 5:00 at RPE 4–5
Fartleks 5:00 at RPE 2–3 10:00 at RPE 3–4 8 × 1:00 at RPE 7–8 / 2:00 at RPE 2–3 15:00 at RPE 3–4	**Foundation Run** 5:00 at RPE 2–3 45:00 at RPE 3–4	**Endurance Run** 5:00 at RPE 2–3 1:20:00 at RPE 3–4 5:00 at RPE 4–5
Hill Repetitions 5:00 at RPE 2–3 10:00 at RPE 3–4 10 × 0:30 uphill at RPE 8–9 / 1:30 at RPE 2–3 15:00 at RPE 2–3	**Foundation Run** 5:00 at RPE 2–3 40:00 at RPE 3–4	**Endurance Run** 5:00 at RPE 2–3 1:10:00 at RPE 3–4 5:00 at RPE 4–5
VO₂max Intervals 5:00 at RPE 2–3 10:00 at RPE 3–4 6 × 2:00* at RPE 7–8 / 2:00 at RPE 2–3 15:00 at RPE 2–3 *Precision Splitting	**Foundation Run** 5:00 at RPE 2–3 45:00 at RPE 3–4	**Endurance Run** 5:00 at RPE 2–3 1:30:00 at RPE 3–4 5:00 at RPE 4–5

	MONDAY	TUESDAY	WEDNESDAY	THURSDAY
5	**Recovery Run** 30:00 at RPE 2–3	**Mini Intervals** 5:00 at RPE 2–3 10:00 at RPE 3–4 40 × (0:30 at 10KP / 0:30 at RPE 2–3) 15:00 at RPE 2–3	**Foundation Run** 5:00 at RPE 2–3 50:00 at RPE 3–4	**Foundation Run** 5:00 at RPE 2–3 50:00 at RPE 3–4
6	Rest	**Progression Run** 5:00 at RPE 2–3 25:00 at RPE 3–4 12:00 at SSP 8:00 at LTP 4:00 at CV 5:00 at RPE 2–3	**Foundation Run** 5:00 at RPE 2–3 45:00 at RPE 3–4	**Foundation Run** 5:00 at RPE 2–3 45:00 at RPE 3–4
7	**Recovery Run** 30:00 at RPE 2–3	**Tempo Run** 5:00 at RPE 2–3 10:00 at RPE 3–4 16:00 at RPE 6 5:00 at RPE 2–3 16:00 at RPE 6 15:00 at RPE 2–3	**Foundation Run** 5:00 at RPE 2–3 50:00 at RPE 3–4	**Foundation Run** 5:00 at RPE 2–3 50:00 at RPE 3–4
8	**Recovery Run** 30:00 at RPE 2–3	**Steady-State Run** 5:00 at RPE 2–3 10:00 at RPE 3–4 40:00 at RPE 5 15:00 at RPE 2–3	**Foundation Run** 5:00 at RPE 2–3 55:00 at RPE 3–4	**Foundation Run** 5:00 at RPE 2–3 55:00 at RPE 3–4
9	Rest	**Fartleks** 5:00 at RPE 2–3 10:00 at RPE 3–4 1:00 at CV, 1:00 at RPE 2–3 2:00 at LTP, 1:00 at RPE 2–3 3:00 at SSP, 1:00 at RPE 2–3 2:00 at LTP, 1:00 at RPE 2–3 1:00 at CV, 1:00 at RPE 2–3 2:00 at LTP, 1:00 at RPE 2–3 1:00 at CV, s1:00 at RPE 2–3 15:00 at RPE 3–4	**Foundation Run** 5:00 at RPE 2–3 45:00 at RPE 3–4	**Foundation Run** 5:00 at RPE 2–3 45:00 at RPE 3–4
10	**Recovery Run** 30:00 at RPE 2–3	**Critical Velocity Intervals** 5:00 at RPE 2–3 10:00 at RPE 3–4 7 × 4:00* at RPE 6–7 / 2:00 at RPE 2–3 15:00 at RPE 2–3 *Precision Splitting*	**Foundation Run** 5:00 at RPE 2–3 55:00 at RPE 3–4	**Foundation Run** 5:00 at RPE 2–3 55:00 at RPE 3–4

How to Run the Perfect Race

FRIDAY	SATURDAY	SUNDAY
Accelerations 5:00 at RPE 2–3 10:00 at RPE 3–4 11:00 acceleration 10:00 at RPE 2–3 6:00 acceleration 15:00 at RPE 2–3	**Foundation Run** 5:00 at RPE 2–3 50:00 at RPE 3–4	**Endurance Run** 5:00 at RPE 2–3 1:40:00 at RPE 3–4 5:00 at RPE 4–5
Speed Intervals 5:00 at RPE 2–3 10:00 at RPE 3–4 8 × 1:00* at RPE 8–9 / 2:00 at RPE 2–3 15:00 at RPE 2–3 *Stretch Intervals*	**Foundation Run** 5:00 at RPE 2–3 45:00 at RPE 3–4	**Endurance Run** 5:00 at RPE 2–3 1:20:00 at RPE 3–4 5:00 at RPE 4–5
5K Pace Intervals 1 km at RPE 2–3 2.5 km at RPE 3–4 6 × (0.8 km at 5KP* / 1:00 rest) 3.5 km at RPE 2–3 *Precision Splitting*	**Foundation Run** 5:00 at RPE 2–3 50:00 at RPE 3–4	**Half-Marathon Pace Run** 1 km at RPE 2–3 2.5 km at RPE 3–4 3 × (3 km at HMP / 1:00 rest) 3.5 km at RPE 2–3
VO₂max Intervals 5:00 at RPE 2–3 10:00 at RPE 3–4 7 × 2:00* at RPE 7–8 / 2:00 at RPE 2–3 15:00 at RPE 2–3 *Precision Splitting*	**Foundation Run** 5:00 at RPE 2–3 55:00 at RPE 3–4	**Endurance Run** 5:00 at RPE 2–3 1:50:00 at RPE 3–4 5:00 at RPE 4–5
Hill Repetitions 5:00 at RPE 2–3 10:00 at RPE 3–4 10 × 1:00 uphill at RPE 8–9* / 2:00 at RPE 2–3 15:00 at RPE 2–3 *Stretch Intervals*	**Foundation Run** 5:00 at RPE 2–3 45:00 at RPE 3–4	**Depletion Run** 5:00 at RPE 2–3 1:10:00 at RPE 3–4 5:00 at RPE 4–5 *No calories before or during*
The Prefontaine 1 km at RPE 2–3 2.5 km at RPE 3–4 ? × 200m at RPE 9 / 200m at RPE 6 1 km at RPE 2–3 2.5 km at RPE 3–4 *(? = Go to failure)*	**Foundation Run** 5:00 at RPE 2–3 55:00 at RPE 3–4	**Half-Marathon Pace Run** 1 km at RPE 2–3 2.5 km at RPE 3–4 2 × (5 km at HMP / 1:00 rest) 3.5 km at RPE 2–3

2 Half-Marathon

	MONDAY	TUESDAY	WEDNESDAY	THURSDAY
11	**Recovery Run** 30:00 at RPE 2–3	**Tempo Run** 5:00 at RPE 2–3 10:00 at RPE 3–4 20:00 at RPE 6 5:00 at RPE 2–3 20:00 at RPE 6 15:00 at RPE 2–3	**Foundation Run** 5:00 at RPE 2–3 55:00 at RPE 3–4	**Foundation Run** 5:00 at RPE 2–3 55:00 at RPE 3–4
12	Rest	**Mini Intervals** 5:00 at RPE 2–3 10:00 at RPE 3–4 40 × (0:30 at CV / 0:30 at RPE 2–3) 15:00 at RPE 2–3	**Foundation Run** 5:00 at RPE 2–3 50:00 at RPE 3–4	**Foundation Run** 5:00 at RPE 2–3 50:00 at RPE 3–4
13	**Recovery Run** 30:00 at RPE 2–3	**Relaxed 10K Time Trial** 1 km at RPE 2–3 2.5 km at RPE 3–4 10 km at 95% effort 3.5 km at RPE 2–3	**Foundation Run** 5:00 at RPE 2–3 55:00 at RPE 3–4	**Foundation Run** 5:00 at RPE 2–3 55:00 at RPE 3–4
14	**Recovery Run** 30:00 at RPE 2–3	**Steady-State Run** 5:00 at RPE 2–3 10:00 at RPE 3–4 50:00 at RPE 5 15:00 at RPE 2–3	**Foundation Run** 5:00 at RPE 2–3 55:00 at RPE 3–4	**Foundation Run** 5:00 at RPE 2–3 50:00 at RPE 3–4
15	Rest	**Fartleks** 5:00 at RPE 2–3 10:00 at RPE 3–4 8 × 1:00 at RPE 7–8 / 2:00 at RPE 2–3 15:00 at RPE 3–4	**Foundation Run** 5:00 at RPE 2–3 40:00 at RPE 3–4	**Foundation Run** 5:00 at RPE 2–3 40:00 at RPE 3–4

How to Run the Perfect Race

FRIDAY	SATURDAY	SUNDAY
Accelerations 5:00 at RPE 2–3 10:00 at RPE 3–4 11:00 acceleration 10:00 at RPE 2–3 6:00 acceleration 10:00 at RPE 2–3 3:00 acceleration 15:00 at RPE 2–3	**Foundation Run** 5:00 at RPE 2–3 55:00 at RPE 3–4	**Endurance Run** 5:00 at RPE 2–3 2:05:00 at RPE 3–4 5:00 at RPE 4–5
Speed Intervals 5:00 at RPE 2–3 5:00 at RPE 3–4 12 × 0:45 at RPE 8–9* / 1:45 at RPE 2–3 10:00 at RPE 2–3 *Stretch Intervals	**Foundation Run** 5:00 at RPE 2–3 50:00 at RPE 3–4	**Depletion Run** 5:00 at RPE 2–3 1:30:00 at RPE 3–4 5:00 at RPE 4–5 *No calories before or during*
VO$_2$max Intervals 5:00 at RPE 2–3 10:00 at RPE 3–4 6 × 2:00 at RPE 7–8* / 2:00 at RPE 2–3 15:00 at RPE 2–3 *Precision Splitting	**Foundation Run** 5:00 at RPE 2–3 55:00 at RPE 3–4	**Half-Marathon Pace Run** 1 km at RPE 2–3 2.5 km at RPE 3–4 13 km at HMP 3.5 km at RPE 2–3
Relaxed 5K Time Trial 1 km at RPE 2–3 1 km at RPE 3–4 5 km at 95% effort 2 km at RPE 2–3	**Foundation Run** 5:00 at RPE 2–3 45:00 at RPE 3–4	**Endurance Run** 5:00 at RPE 2–3 1:10:00 at RPE 3–4 5:00 at RPE 4–5
Fast Finish Run 5:00 at RPE 2–3 20:00 at RPE 3–4 10:00 at RPE 6	**Foundation Run** 5:00 at RPE 2–3 15:00 at RPE 3–4	**Half-Marathon Race**

Half-Marathon

2

Half-Marathon

This plan was designed for serious competitive runners seeking the absolute limit of their potential at the half-marathon distance. Before starting the plan, be sure to build your training to the point where you're comfortably able to run 9 times per week for up to 80 minutes.

	MONDAY	TUESDAY	WEDNESDAY	THURSDAY
1	**Recovery Run** 40:00 at RPE 2–3	**Progression Run** 5:00 at RPE 2–3 35:00 at RPE 3–4 8:00 at SSP 4:00 at LTP 2:00 at CV 5:00 at RPE 2–3 **Recovery Run** 20:00 at RPE 2–3	**Foundation Run** 5:00 at RPE 2–3 55:00 at RPE 3–4	**Foundation Run** 5:00 at RPE 2–3 55:00 at RPE 3–4
2	**Recovery Run** 40:00 at RPE 2–3	**Progression Run** 5:00 at RPE 2–3 35:00 at RPE 3–4 4:00 at LTP 2:00 at CV 1:00 at MAS 5:00 at RPE 2–3 **Recovery Run** 20:00 at RPE 2–3	**Foundation Run** 5:00 at RPE 2–3 55:00 at RPE 3–4	**Foundation Run** 5:00 at RPE 2–3 55:00 at RPE 3–4
3	Rest	**Fartleks** 5:00 at RPE 2–3 15:00 at RPE 3–4 1:00 at CV, 1:00 at RPE 2–3 2:00 at LTP, 1:00 at RPE 2–3 3:00 at SSP, 1:00 at RPE 2–3 2:00 at LTP, 1:00 at RPE 2–3 1:00 at CV, 1:00 at RPE 2–3 2:00 at LTP, 1:00 at RPE 2–3 3:00 at SSP, 1:00 at RPE 2–3 20:00 at RPE 3–4 **Recovery Run** 20:00 at RPE 2–3	**Foundation Run** 5:00 at RPE 2–3 45:00 at RPE 3–4	**Foundation Run** 5:00 at RPE 2–3 45:00 at RPE 3–4

LEVEL 3

SSP   Steady-State Pace
LTP   Lactate Threshold Pace
CV   Critical Velocity
MAS   Maximal Aerobic Speed

5KP   5K Pace
10KP 10K Pace
HMP Half-Marathon Pace
MP   Marathon Pace

FRIDAY	SATURDAY	SUNDAY
Fartleks 5:00 at RPE 2–3 15:00 at RPE 3–4 10 × 0:20 at RPE 8–9 / 1:40 at RPE 2–3 20:00 at RPE 3–4 --- **Recovery Run** 20:00 at RPE 2–3	**Foundation Run** 5:00 at RPE 2–3 55:00 at RPE 3–4	**Endurance Run** 5:00 at RPE 2–3 1:10:00 at RPE 3–4 5:00 at RPE 4–5
Fartleks 5:00 at RPE 2–3 10:00 at RPE 3–4 8 × 1:00 at RPE 7–8 / 2:00 at RPE 2–3 15:00 at RPE 3–4 --- **Recovery Run** 20:00 at RPE 2–3	**Foundation Run** 5:00 at RPE 2–3 55:00 at RPE 3–4	**Endurance Run** 5:00 at RPE 2–3 1:30:00 at RPE 3–4 5:00 at RPE 4–5
Hill Repetitions 5:00 at RPE 2–3 15:00 at RPE 3–4 12 × 0:30 uphill at RPE 8–9 / 1:30 at RPE 2–3 20:00 at RPE 2–3 --- **Recovery Run** 20:00 at RPE 2–3	**Foundation Run** 5:00 at RPE 2–3 45:00 at RPE 3–4	**Endurance Run** 5:00 at RPE 2–3 1:20:00 at RPE 3–4 5:00 at RPE 4–5

3 Half-Marathon

	MONDAY	TUESDAY	WEDNESDAY	THURSDAY
4	**Recovery Run** 40:00 at RPE 2–3	**Critical Velocity Intervals** 5:00 at RPE 2–3 15:00 at RPE 3–4 7 × 4:00* at RPE 6–7 / 2:00 at RPE 2–3 20:00 at RPE 2–3 *Precision Splitting* **Recovery Run** 25:00 at RPE 2–3	**Foundation Run** 5:00 at RPE 2–3 55:00 at RPE 3–4	**Foundation Run** 5:00 at RPE 2–3 1:00:00 at RPE 3–4
5	**Recovery Run** 40:00 at RPE 2–3	**Mini Intervals** 5:00 at RPE 2–3 15:00 at RPE 3–4 50 × (0:30 at 10KP / 0:30 at RPE 2–3) 20:00 at RPE 2–3 **Recovery Run** 25:00 at RPE 2–3	**Foundation Run** 5:00 at RPE 2–3 55:00 at RPE 3–4	**Foundation Run** 5:00 at RPE 2–3 1:00:00 at RPE 3–4
6	Rest	**Progression Run** 5:00 at RPE 2–3 30:00 at RPE 3–4 12:00 at SSP 8:00 at LTP 4:00 at CV 5:00 at RPE 2–3 **Recovery Run** 20:00 at RPE 2–3	**Foundation Run** 5:00 at RPE 2–3 50:00 at RPE 3–4	**Foundation Run** 5:00 at RPE 2–3 50:00 at RPE 3–4
7	**Recovery Run** 40:00 at RPE 2–3	**Tempo Run** 5:00 at RPE 2–3 15:00 at RPE 3–4 18:00 at RPE 6 5:00 at RPE 2–3 18:00 at RPE 6 20:00 at RPE 2–3 **Recovery Run** 30:00 at RPE 2–3	**Foundation Run** 5:00 at RPE 2–3 55:00 at RPE 3–4	**Foundation Run** 5:00 at RPE 2–3 1:05:00 at RPE 3–4
8	**Recovery Run** 40:00 at RPE 2–3	**Steady-State Run** 5:00 at RPE 2–3 15:00 at RPE 3–4 45:00 at RPE 5 20:00 at RPE 2–3 **Recovery Run** 30:00 at RPE 2–3	**Foundation Run** 5:00 at RPE 2–3 55:00 at RPE 3–4	**Foundation Run** 5:00 at RPE 2–3 1:05:00 at RPE 3–4

How to Run the Perfect Race

FRIDAY	SATURDAY	SUNDAY
VO₂max Intervals 5:00 at RPE 2–3 15:00 at RPE 3–4 7 × 2:00* at RPE 7–8 / 2:00 at RPE 2–3 20:00 at RPE 2–3 *Precision Splitting*<hr>**Recovery Run** 25:00 at RPE 2–3	**Foundation Run** 5:00 at RPE 2–3 55:00 at RPE 3–4	**Endurance Run** 5:00 at RPE 2–3 1:50:00 at RPE 3–4 5:00 at RPE 4–5
Accelerations 5:00 at RPE 2–3 15:00 at RPE 3–4 11:00 acceleration 10:00 at RPE 2–3 6:00 acceleration 10:00 at RPE 2–3 11:00 acceleration 20:00 at RPE 2–3<hr>**Recovery Run** 25:00 at RPE 2–3	**Foundation Run** 5:00 at RPE 2–3 55:00 at RPE 3–4	**Marathon Pace Run** 1 km (0.6 mile) at RPE 2–3 2 km (1.2 miles) at RPE 3–4 5 × 1.5 km (0.9 mile) at MP / 1.5 km (0.9 mile) at RPE 3–4 2 km (1.2 miles) at RPE 2–3
Speed Intervals 5:00 at RPE 2–3 15:00 at RPE 3–4 10 × 1:00* at RPE 8–9 / 2:00 at RPE 2–3 20:00 at RPE 2–3 *Stretch Intervals*<hr>**Recovery Run** 20:00 at RPE 2–3	**Foundation Run** 5:00 at RPE 2–3 50:00 at RPE 3–4	**Depletion Run** 5:00 at RPE 2–3 1:15:00 at RPE 3–4 *No calories before or during*
5K Pace Intervals 1 km at RPE 2–3 4 km at RPE 3–4 6 × (0.8 km at 5KP* / 1:00 rest) 5 km at RPE 2–3 *Precision Splitting*<hr>**Recovery Run** 30:00 at RPE 2–3	**Foundation Run** 5:00 at RPE 2–3 55:00 at RPE 3–4	**Half-Marathon Pace Run** 1 km at RPE 2–3 4 km at RPE 3–4 3 × (3 km at HMP / 1:00 rest) 5 km at RPE 2–3
VO₂max Intervals 5:00 at RPE 2–3 15:00 at RPE 3–4 8 × 2:00* at RPE 7–8 / 2:00 at RPE 2–3 20:00 at RPE 2–3 *Precision Splitting*<hr>**Recovery Run** 30:00 at RPE 2–3	**Foundation Run** 5:00 at RPE 2–3 55:00 at RPE 3–4	**Endurance Run** 5:00 at RPE 2–3 2:05:00 at RPE 3–4 5:00 at RPE 4–5

3 Half-Marathon

	MONDAY	TUESDAY	WEDNESDAY	THURSDAY
9	Rest	**Fartleks** 5:00 at RPE 2–3 15:00 at RPE 3–4 1:00 at CV, 1:00 at RPE 2–3 2:00 at LTP, 1:00 at RPE 2–3 3:00 at SSP, 1:00 at RPE 2–3 2:00 at LTP, 1:00 at RPE 2–3 1:00 at CV, 1:00 at RPE 2–3 2:00 at LTP, 1:00 at RPE 2–3 3:00 at SSP, 1:00 at RPE 2–3 2:00 at LTP, 1:00 at RPE 2–3 1:00 at CV, 1:00 at RPE 2–3 20:00 at RPE 3–4 **Recovery Run** 25:00 at RPE 2–3	**Foundation Run** 5:00 at RPE 2–3 55:00 at RPE 3–4	**Foundation Run** 5:00 at RPE 2–3 55:00 at RPE 3–4
10	**Recovery Run** 40:00 at RPE 2–3	**Critical Velocity Intervals** 5:00 at RPE 2–3 15:00 at RPE 3–4 8 × 4:00* at RPE 6–7 / 2:00 at RPE 2–3 20:00 at RPE 2–3 *Precision Splitting* **Recovery Run** 35:00 at RPE 2–3	**Foundation Run** 5:00 at RPE 2–3 55:00 at RPE 3–4	**Foundation Run** 5:00 at RPE 2–3 1:10:00 at RPE 3–4
11	**Recovery Run** 40:00 at RPE 2–3	**Tempo Run** 5:00 at RPE 2–3 15:00 at RPE 3–4 22:00 at RPE 6 5:00 at RPE 2–3 22:00 at RPE 6 20:00 at RPE 2–3 **Recovery Run** 35:00 at RPE 2–3	**Foundation Run** 5:00 at RPE 2–3 55:00 at RPE 3–4	**Foundation Run** 5:00 at RPE 2–3 1:10:00 at RPE 3–4
12	Rest	**Mini Intervals** 5:00 at RPE 2–3 15:00 at RPE 3–4 50 × (0:30 at CV / 0:30 at RPE 2–3) 20:00 at RPE 2–3 **Recovery Run** 30:00 at RPE 2–3	**Foundation Run** 5:00 at RPE 2–3 55:00 at RPE 3–4	**Foundation Run** 5:00 at RPE 2–3 1:00:00 at RPE 3–4

How to Run the Perfect Race

FRIDAY	SATURDAY	SUNDAY
Hill Repetitions 5:00 at RPE 2–3 15:00 at RPE 3–4 10 × 1:00 uphill at RPE 8–9* / 2:00 at RPE 2–3 20:00 at RPE 2–3 *Stretch Intervals **Recovery Run** 25:00 at RPE 2–3	**Foundation Run** 5:00 at RPE 2–3 55:00 at RPE 3–4	**Depletion Run** 5:00 at RPE 2–3 1:35:00 at RPE 3–4 *No calories before or during*
The Prefontaine 1 km at RPE 2–3 4 km at RPE 3–4 ? × 200m at RPE 9 / 200m at RPE 6 1 km at RPE 2–3 4 km at RPE 3–4 (? = Go to failure) **Recovery Run** 35:00 at RPE 2–3	**Foundation Run** 5:00 at RPE 2–3 55:00 at RPE 3–4	**Half-Marathon Pace Run** 1 km at RPE 2–3 4 km at RPE 3–4 2 × (5 km at HMP / 1:00 rest) 5 km at RPE 2–3
Accelerations 5:00 at RPE 2–3 15:00 at RPE 3–4 11:00 acceleration 10:00 at RPE 2–3 6:00 acceleration 10:00 at RPE 2–3 3:00 acceleration 20:00 at RPE 2–3 **Recovery Run** 35:00 at RPE 2–3	**Foundation Run** 5:00 at RPE 2–3 55:00 at RPE 3–4	**Endurance Run** 5:00 at RPE 2–3 2:25:00 at RPE 3–4 5:00 at RPE 4–5
Speed Intervals 5:00 at RPE 2–3 15:00 at RPE 3–4 12 × 0:45 at RPE 8–9* / 1:45 at RPE 2–3 20:00 at RPE 2–3 *Stretch Intervals **Recovery Run** 30:00 at RPE 2–3	**Foundation Run** 5:00 at RPE 2–3 55:00 at RPE 3–4	**Depletion Run** 5:00 at RPE 2–3 1:55:00 at RPE 3–4 *No calories before or during*

3 Half-Marathon

	MONDAY	TUESDAY	WEDNESDAY	THURSDAY
13	**Recovery Run** 40:00 at RPE 2–3	**Relaxed 10K Time Trial** 1 km at RPE 2–3 4 km at RPE 3–4 10 km at 95% effort 5 km at RPE 2–3 — **Recovery Run** 35:00 at RPE 2–3	**Foundation Run** 5:00 at RPE 2–3 55:00 at RPE 3–4	**Foundation Run** 5:00 at RPE 2–3 1:10:00 at RPE 3–4
14	**Recovery Run** 40:00 at RPE 2–3	**Steady-State Run** 5:00 at RPE 2–3 15:00 at RPE 3–4 1:00:00 at RPE 5 20:00 at RPE 2–3 — **Recovery Run** 30:00 at RPE 2–3	**Foundation Run** 5:00 at RPE 2–3 55:00 at RPE 3–4	**Foundation Run** 5:00 at RPE 2–3 55:00 at RPE 3–4
15	Rest	**Fartleks** 5:00 at RPE 2–3 15:00 at RPE 3–4 10 × 1:00 at RPE 7–8 / 2:00 at RPE 2–3 20:00 at RPE 3–4	**Foundation Run** 5:00 at RPE 2–3 40:00 at RPE 3–4	**Foundation Run** 5:00 at RPE 2–3 40:00 at RPE 3–4

FRIDAY	**SATURDAY**	**SUNDAY**
VO$_2$max Intervals 5:00 at RPE 2–3 15:00 at RPE 3–4 7 × 2:00 at RPE 7–8* / 2:00 at RPE 2–3 20:00 at RPE 2–3 *Precision Splitting **Recovery Run** 35:00 at RPE 2–3	**Foundation Run** 5:00 at RPE 2–3 55:00 at RPE 3–4	**Half-Marathon Pace Run** 1 km at RPE 2–3 4 km at RPE 3–4 13 km at HMP 5 km at RPE 2–3
Relaxed 5K Time Trial 1 km at RPE 2–3 4 km at RPE 3–4 5 km at 95% effort 5 km at RPE 2–3 **Recovery Run** 30:00 at RPE 2–3	**Foundation Run** 5:00 at RPE 2–3 55:00 at RPE 3–4	**Endurance Run** 5:00 at RPE 2–3 1:10:00 at RPE 3–4 5:00 at RPE 4–5
Fast Finish Run 5:00 at RPE 2–3 20:00 at RPE 3–4 10:00 at RPE 6	**Foundation Run** 5:00 at RPE 2–3 15:00 at RPE 3–4	## Half-Marathon Race

3 Half-Marathon

12

Marathon Training Plans

The four training plans presented in this chapter are designed to help runners master the art of pacing and find their limit at the marathon distance. The various levels cover the needs of everyone from first-timers to elites. Refer back to Chapter 6 for details on the RPE-based intensity scale used throughout the plans and for full explanations of certain terms and workout types. Online versions of the plans are available for separate purchase on the 80/20 Endurance web site. Additionally, device-compatible free versions of the individual workouts can be found at https://www.8020endurance.com.

Marathon

This plan is appropriate for beginning runners preparing for their first marathon event and for more experienced runners who need or prefer a relatively low-volume training program for any reason. Before starting the plan, be sure to build your training to the point where you're comfortably able to run 5 days a week for up to 10 km.

	MONDAY	TUESDAY	WEDNESDAY	THURSDAY
1	Rest	**Progression Run** 5:00 at RPE 2–3 10:00 at RPE 3–4 8:00 at SSP 4:00 at LTP 2:00 at CV 5:00 at RPE 2–3	**Foundation Run** 5:00 at RPE 2–3 25:00 at RPE 3–4	Rest
2	Rest	**Progression Run** 5:00 at RPE 2–3 20:00 at RPE 3–4 4:00 at LTP 2:00 at CV 1:00 at MAS 5:00 at RPE 2–3	**Foundation Run** 5:00 at RPE 2–3 30:00 at RPE 3–4	Rest
3	Rest	**Progression Run** 5:00 at RPE 2–3 10:00 at RPE 3–4 8:00 at SSP 4:00 at LTP 2:00 at CV 5:00 at RPE 2–3	**Foundation Run** 5:00 at RPE 2–3 25:00 at RPE 3–4	Rest
4	Rest	**Mini Intervals** 5:00 at RPE 2–3 5:00 at RPE 3–4 20 × (0:30 at 10KP / 0:30 at RPE 2–3) 10:00 at RPE 2–3	**Foundation Run** 5:00 at RPE 2–3 30:00 at RPE 3–4	Rest
5	Rest	**Critical Velocity Intervals** 5:00 at RPE 2–3 5:00 at RPE 3–4 4 × 4:00 at RPE 6–7* / 2:00 at RPE 2–3 10:00 at RPE 2–3 *Precision Splitting	**Foundation Run** 5:00 at RPE 2–3 35:00 at RPE 3–4	Rest

LEVEL 0

SSP Steady-State Pace
LTP Lactate Threshold Pace
CV   Critical Velocity
MAS Maximal Aerobic Speed

5KP 5K Pace

FRIDAY	SATURDAY	SUNDAY
Fartleks 5:00 at RPE 2–3 5:00 at RPE 3–4 4 × 1:00 at RPE 7–8 / 2:00 at RPE 2–3 10:00 at RPE 3–4	**Foundation Run** 5:00 at RPE 2–3 25:00 at RPE 3–4	**Long Run with Fast Finish** 1 km at RPE 2–3 8 km at RPE 3–4 1 km at RPE 4–5
Fartleks 5:00 at RPE 2–3 5:00 at RPE 3–4 6 × 0:20 at RPE 8–9 / 1:40 at RPE 2–3 10:00 at RPE 3–4	**Foundation Run** 5:00 at RPE 2–3 30:00 at RPE 3–4	**Long Run with Fast Finish** 1 km at RPE 2–3 9 km at RPE 3–4 1 km at RPE 4–5
Fartleks 5:00 at RPE 2–3 5:00 at RPE 3–4 6 × 1:00 at RPE 7–8 / 2:00 at RPE 2–3 10:00 at RPE 3–4	**Foundation Run** 5:00 at RPE 2–3 25:00 at RPE 3–4	**Long Run with Fast Finish** 1 km at RPE 2–3 8 km at RPE 3–4 1 km at RPE 4–5
Hill Repetitions 5:00 at RPE 2–3 5:00 at RPE 3–4 8 × 0:30 uphill at RPE 8–9* / 1:30 at RPE 2–3 10:00 at RPE 2–3 *Stretch Intervals	**Foundation Run** 5:00 at RPE 2–3 30:00 at RPE 3–4	**Long Run with Fast Finish** 1 km at RPE 2–3 11 km at RPE 3–4 1 km at RPE 4–5
Accelerations 5:00 at RPE 2–3 5:00 at RPE 3–4 11:00 acceleration 10:00 at RPE 2–3 3:00 acceleration 10:00 at RPE 2–3	**Foundation Run** 5:00 at RPE 2–3 35:00 at RPE 3–4	**Long Run with Fast Finish** 1 km at RPE 2–3 13 km at RPE 3–4 1 km at RPE 4–5

	MONDAY	TUESDAY	WEDNESDAY	THURSDAY
6	Rest	**Fartleks** 5:00 at RPE 2–3 5:00 at RPE 3–4 1:00 at CV, 1:00 at RPE 2–3 2:00 at LTP, 1:00 at RPE 2–3 3:00 at SSP, 1:00 at RPE 2–3 2:00 at LTP, 1:00 at RPE 2–3 1:00 at CV, 1:00 at RPE 2–3 10:00 at RPE 3–4	**Foundation Run** 5:00 at RPE 2–3 30:00 at RPE 3–4	Rest
7	Rest	**Steady-State Run** 5:00 at RPE 2–3 5:00 at RPE 3–4 35:00 at RPE 5 10:00 at RPE 2–3	**Foundation Run** 5:00 at RPE 2–3 35:00 at RPE 3–4	Rest
8	Rest	**Tempo Run** 5:00 at RPE 2–3 5:00 at RPE 3–4 12:00 at RPE 6 5:00 at RPE 2–3 12:00 at RPE 6 10:00 at RPE 2–3	**Foundation Run** 5:00 at RPE 2–3 40:00 at RPE 3–4	Rest
9	Rest	**Fartleks** 5:00 at RPE 2–3 5:00 at RPE 3–4 1:00 at CV, 1:00 at RPE 2–3 2:00 at LTP, 1:00 at RPE 2–3 3:00 at SSP, 1:00 at RPE 2–3 2:00 at LTP, 1:00 at RPE 2–3 1:00 at CV, 1:00 at RPE 2–3 2:00 at LTP, 1:00 at RPE 2–3 1:00 at CV, 1:00 at RPE 2–3 10:00 at RPE 3–4	**Foundation Run** 5:00 at RPE 2–3 35:00 at RPE 3–4	Rest
10	Rest	**Mini Intervals** 5:00 at RPE 2–3 5:00 at RPE 3–4 20 × (0:30 at CV / 0:30 at RPE 2–3) 10:00 at RPE 2–3	**Foundation Run** 5:00 at RPE 2–3 40:00 at RPE 3–4	Rest
11	Rest	**Critical Velocity Intervals** 5:00 at RPE 2–3 5:00 at RPE 3–4 5 × 4:00 at RPE 6–7* / 2:00 at RPE 2–3 10:00 at RPE 2–3 *Precision Splitting*	**Foundation Run** 5:00 at RPE 2–3 45:00 at RPE 3–4	Rest

FRIDAY	SATURDAY	SUNDAY
Speed Intervals 5:00 at RPE 2–3 5:00 at RPE 3–4 6 × 0:45 at RPE 8–9* / 1:45 at RPE 2–3 10:00 at RPE 2–3 *Stretch Intervals*	**Foundation Run** 5:00 at RPE 2–3 30:00 at RPE 3–4	**Long Run with Fast Finish** 1 km at RPE 2–3 11 km at RPE 3–4 1 km at RPE 4–5
VO₂max Intervals 5:00 at RPE 2–3 5:00 at RPE 3–4 4 × 2:00 at RPE 7–8* / 2:00 at RPE 2–3 10:00 at RPE 2–3 *Precision Splitting*	**Foundation Run** 5:00 at RPE 2–3 35:00 at RPE 3–4	**Long Run with Fast Finish** 1 km at RPE 2–3 15 km at RPE 3–4 1 km at RPE 4–5
5K Pace Intervals 1 km at RPE 2–3 1 km at RPE 3–4 6 × (0.8 km at 5KP* / 1:00 rest) 2 km at RPE 2–3 *Precision Splitting*	**Foundation Run** 5:00 at RPE 2–3 40:00 at RPE 3–4	**Long Run with Fast Finish** 1 km at RPE 2–3 17 km at RPE 3–4 1 km at RPE 4–5
Hill Repetitions 5:00 at RPE 2–3 5:00 at RPE 3–4 6 × 1:00 uphill at RPE 8–9* / 2:00 at RPE 2–3 10:00 at RPE 2–3 *Stretch Intervals*	**Foundation Run** 5:00 at RPE 2–3 35:00 at RPE 3–4	**Long Run with Fast Finish** 1 km at RPE 2–3 13 km at RPE 3–4 1 km at RPE 4–5
5K Pace Intervals 1 km at RPE 2–3 1 km at RPE 3–4 8 × (0.6 km at 5KP* / 1:00 rest) 2 km at RPE 2–3 *Precision Splitting*	**Foundation Run** 5:00 at RPE 2–3 40:00 at RPE 3–4	**Long Run with Fast Finish** 1 km at RPE 2–3 19 km at RPE 3–4 1 km at RPE 4–5
5K Pace Intervals 1 km at RPE 2–3 1 km at RPE 3–4 8 × (0.6 km at 5KP* / 1:00 rest) 2 km at RPE 2–3 *Precision Splitting*	**Foundation Run** 5:00 at RPE 2–3 45:00 at RPE 3–4	**Long Run with Fast Finish** 1 km at RPE 2–3 21 km at RPE 3–4 1 km at RPE 4–5

Marathon

	MONDAY	TUESDAY	WEDNESDAY	THURSDAY
12	Rest	**Fartleks** 5:00 at RPE 2–3 5:00 at RPE 3–4 1:00 at CV, 1:00 at RPE 2–3 2:00 at LTP, 1:00 at RPE 2–3 3:00 at SSP, 1:00 at RPE 2–3 2:00 at LTP, 1:00 at RPE 2–3 1:00 at CV, 1:00 at RPE 2–3 2:00 at LTP, 1:00 at RPE 2–3 1:00 at CV, 1:00 at RPE 2–3 2:00 at LTP, 1:00 at RPE 2–3 3:00 at SSP, 1:00 at RPE 2–3 10:00 at RPE 3–4	**Foundation Run** 5:00 at RPE 2–3 40:00 at RPE 3–4	Rest
13	Rest	**Steady-State Run** 5:00 at RPE 2–3 5:00 at RPE 3–4 40:00 at RPE 5 10:00 at RPE 2–3	**Foundation Run** 5:00 at RPE 2–3 45:00 at RPE 3–4	Rest
14	Rest	**Tempo Run** 5:00 at RPE 2–3 5:00 at RPE 3–4 14:00 at RPE 6 5:00 at RPE 2–3 14:00 at RPE 6 10:00 at RPE 2–3	**Foundation Run** 5:00 at RPE 2–3 50:00 at RPE 3–4	Rest
15	Rest	**Progression Run** 5:00 at RPE 2–3 15:00 at RPE 3–4 12:00 at SSP 6:00 at LTP 3:00 at CV 5:00 at RPE 2–3	**Foundation Run** 5:00 at RPE 2–3 40:00 at RPE 3–4	Rest
16	Rest	**Steady-State Run** 5:00 at RPE 2–3 5:00 at RPE 3–4 50:00 at RPE 5 10:00 at RPE 2–3	**Foundation Run** 5:00 at RPE 2–3 50:00 at RPE 3–4	Rest
17	Rest	**Relaxed 10K Time Trial** 1 km at RPE 2–3 1 km at RPE 3–4 10 km at 95% effort 2 km at RPE 2–3	**Foundation Run** 5:00 at RPE 2–3 40:00 at RPE 3–4	Rest
18	Rest	**Fartleks** 5:00 at RPE 2–3 5:00 at RPE 3–4 6 × 1:00 at RPE 7–8 / 2:00 at RPE 2–3 10:00 at RPE 3–4	**Foundation Run** 5:00 at RPE 2–3 40:00 at RPE 3–4	Rest

How to Run the Perfect Race

FRIDAY	SATURDAY	SUNDAY
Speed Intervals 5:00 at RPE 2–3 5:00 at RPE 3–4 8 × 0:45 at RPE 8–9* / 1:45 at RPE 2–3 10:00 at RPE 2–3 *Stretch Intervals*	**Foundation Run** 5:00 at RPE 2–3 40:00 at RPE 3–4	**Long Run with Fast Finish** 1 km at RPE 2–3 15 km at RPE 3–4 1 km at RPE 4–5
Accelerations 5:00 at RPE 2–3 5:00 at RPE 3–4 11:00 acceleration 10:00 at RPE 2–3 6:00 acceleration 10:00 at RPE 2–3	**Foundation Run** 5:00 at RPE 2–3 45:00 at RPE 3–4	**Long Run with Fast Finish** 1 km at RPE 2–3 23 km at RPE 3–4 1 km at RPE 4–5
Hill Repetitions 5:00 at RPE 2–3 5:00 at RPE 3–4 5 × 2:00 uphill at RPE 7–8* / 1:00 at RPE 2–3 10:00 at RPE 2–3 *Precision Splitting*	**Foundation Run** 5:00 at RPE 2–3 50:00 at RPE 3–4	**Long Run with Fast Finish** 1 km at RPE 2–3 25 km at RPE 3–4 1 km at RPE 4–5
Speed Intervals 5:00 at RPE 2–3 5:00 at RPE 3–4 10 × 0:45 at RPE 8–9* / 1:45 at RPE 2–3 10:00 at RPE 2–3 *Stretch Intervals*	**Foundation Run** 5:00 at RPE 2–3 40:00 at RPE 3–4	**Long Run with Fast Finish** 1 km at RPE 2–3 17 km at RPE 3–4 1 km at RPE 4–5
Relaxed 5K Time Trial 1 km at RPE 2–3 1 km at RPE 3–4 5 km at 95% effort 2 km at RPE 2–3	**Foundation Run** 5:00 at RPE 2–3 50:00 at RPE 3–4	**Long Run with Fast Finish** 1 km at RPE 2–3 27 km at RPE 3–4 1 km at RPE 4–5
VO$_2$max Intervals 5:00 at RPE 2–3 5:00 at RPE 3–4 4 × 2:00 at RPE 7–8* / 2:00 at RPE 2–3 10:00 at RPE 2–3 *Precision Splitting*	**Foundation Run** 5:00 at RPE 2–3 40:00 at RPE 3–4	**Long Run with Fast Finish** 1 km at RPE 2–3 15 km at RPE 3–4 1 km at RPE 4–5
Fast Finish Run 5:00 at RPE 2–3 15:00 at RPE 3–4 10:00 at RPE 6	**Foundation Run** 5:00 at RPE 2–3 15:00 at RPE 3–4	**Marathon Race**

Marathon

Marathon

This plan is designed for runners who are ready to take their training load up a notch in order to improve their marathon time. Before starting the plan, be sure to build your training to the point where you're comfortably able to run 6 days a week for up to 12 km.

	MONDAY	TUESDAY	WEDNESDAY	THURSDAY
1	Rest	**Progression Run** 5:00 at RPE 2–3 15:00 at RPE 3–4 8:00 at SSP 4:00 at LTP 2:00 at CV 5:00 at RPE 2–3	**Foundation Run** 5:00 at RPE 2–3 25:00 at RPE 3–4	**Foundation Run** 5:00 at RPE 2–3 25:00 at RPE 3–4
2	Rest	**Progression Run** 5:00 at RPE 2–3 25:00 at RPE 3–4 4:00 at LTP 2:00 at CV 1:00 at MAS 5:00 at RPE 2–3	**Foundation Run** 5:00 at RPE 2–3 30:00 at RPE 3–4	**Foundation Run** 5:00 at RPE 2–3 30:00 at RPE 3–4
3	Rest	**Progression Run** 5:00 at RPE 2–3 10:00 at RPE 3–4 8:00 at SSP 4:00 at LTP 2:00 at CV 5:00 at RPE 2–3	**Foundation Run** 5:00 at RPE 2–3 25:00 at RPE 3–4	**Foundation Run** 5:00 at RPE 2–3 25:00 at RPE 3–4
4	Rest	**Mini Intervals** 5:00 at RPE 2–3 5:00 at RPE 3–4 30 × (0:30 at 10KP / 0:30 at RPE 2–3 10:00 at RPE 2–3	**Foundation Run** 5:00 at RPE 2–3 30:00 at RPE 3–4	**Foundation Run** 5:00 at RPE 2–3 30:00 at RPE 3–4
5	Rest	**Critical Velocity Intervals** 5:00 at RPE 2–3 5:00 at RPE 3–4 5 × 4:00 at RPE 6–7* / 2:00 at RPE 2–3 10:00 at RPE 2–3 *Precision Splitting*	**Foundation Run** 5:00 at RPE 2–3 35:00 at RPE 3–4	**Foundation Run** 5:00 at RPE 2–3 35:00 at RPE 3–4

How to Run the Perfect Race

LEVEL

SSP   Steady-State Pace
LTP   Lactate Threshold Pace
CV   Critical Velocity
MAS Maximal Aerobic Speed

5KP 5K Pace
10KP 10K Pace
MP   Marathon Pace

FRIDAY	SATURDAY	SUNDAY
Fartleks 5:00 at RPE 2–3 5:00 at RPE 3–4 6 × 1:00 at RPE 7–8 / 2:00 at RPE 2–3 10:00 at RPE 3–4	**Foundation Run** 5:00 at RPE 2–3 25:00 at RPE 3–4	**Long Run with Fast Finish** 1 km at RPE 2–3 11 km at RPE 3–4 1 km at RPE 4–5
Fartleks 5:00 at RPE 2–3 5:00 at RPE 3–4 6 × 0:20 at RPE 8–9 / 1:40 at RPE 2–3 10:00 at RPE 3–4	**Foundation Run** 5:00 at RPE 2–3 30:00 at RPE 3–4	**Long Run with Fast Finish** 1 km at RPE 2–3 13 km at RPE 3–4 1 km at RPE 4–5
Fartleks 5:00 at RPE 2–3 5:00 at RPE 3–4 6 × 1:00 at RPE 7–8 / 2:00 at RPE 2–3 10:00 at RPE 3–4	**Foundation Run** 5:00 at RPE 2–3 25:00 at RPE 3–4	**Long Run with Fast Finish** 1 km at RPE 2–3 11 km at RPE 3–4 1 km at RPE 4–5
Hill Repetitions 5:00 at RPE 2–3 5:00 at RPE 3–4 8 × 0:30 uphill at RPE 8–9* / 1:30 at RPE 2–3 10:00 at RPE 2–3 *Stretch Intervals*	**Foundation Run** 5:00 at RPE 2–3 30:00 at RPE 3–4	**Long Run with Fast Finish** 1 km at RPE 2–3 15 km at RPE 3–4 1 km at RPE 4–5
Accelerations 5:00 at RPE 2–3 5:00 at RPE 3–4 11:00 acceleration 10:00 at RPE 2–3 6:00 acceleration 10:00 at RPE 2–3	**Foundation Run** 5:00 at RPE 2–3 35:00 at RPE 3–4	**Long Run with Fast Finish** 1 km at RPE 2–3 17 km at RPE 3–4 1 km at RPE 4–5

Marathon

1

	MONDAY	TUESDAY	WEDNESDAY	THURSDAY
6	Rest	**Fartleks** 5:00 at RPE 2–3 5:00 at RPE 3–4 1:00 at CV, 1:00 at RPE 2–3 2:00 at LTP, 1:00 at RPE 2–3 3:00 at SSP, 1:00 at RPE 2–3 2:00 at LTP, 1:00 at RPE 2–3 1:00 at CV, 1:00 at RPE 2–3 2:00 at LTP, 1:00 at RPE 2–3 3:00 at SSP, 1:00 at RPE 2–3 10:00 at RPE 3–4	**Foundation Run** 5:00 at RPE 2–3 30:00 at RPE 3–4	**Foundation Run** 5:00 at RPE 2–3 30:00 at RPE 3–4
7	Rest	**Steady-State Run** 5:00 at RPE 2–3 5:00 at RPE 3–4 40:00 at RPE 5 10:00 at RPE 2–3	**Foundation Run** 5:00 at RPE 2–3 35:00 at RPE 3–4	**Foundation Run** 5:00 at RPE 2–3 35:00 at RPE 3–4
8	Rest	**Tempo Run** 5:00 at RPE 2–3 5:00 at RPE 3–4 14:00 at RPE 6 5:00 at RPE 2–3 14:00 at RPE 6 10:00 at RPE 2–3	**Foundation Run** 5:00 at RPE 2–3 40:00 at RPE 3–4	**Foundation Run** 5:00 at RPE 2–3 40:00 at RPE 3–4
9	Rest	**Progression Run** 5:00 at RPE 2–3 20:00 at RPE 3–4 8:00 at LTP 4:00 at CV 2:00 at MAS 5:00 at RPE 2–3	**Foundation Run** 5:00 at RPE 2–3 35:00 at RPE 3–4	**Foundation Run** 5:00 at RPE 2–3 35:00 at RPE 3–4
10	Rest	**Mini Intervals** 5:00 at RPE 2–3 5:00 at RPE 3–4 30 × (0:30 at CV / 0:30 at RPE 2–3) 10:00 at RPE 2–3	**Foundation Run** 5:00 at RPE 2–3 40:00 at RPE 3–4	**Foundation Run** 5:00 at RPE 2–3 40:00 at RPE 3–4
11	Rest	**Critical Velocity Intervals** 5:00 at RPE 2–3 5:00 at RPE 3–4 6 × 4:00 at RPE 6–7* / 2:00 at RPE 2–3 10:00 at RPE 2–3 *Precision Splitting*	**Foundation Run** 5:00 at RPE 2–3 45:00 at RPE 3–4	**Foundation Run** 5:00 at RPE 2–3 45:00 at RPE 3–4

FRIDAY	SATURDAY	SUNDAY
Speed Intervals 5:00 at RPE 2–3 5:00 at RPE 3–4 8 × 0:45 at RPE 8–9* / 1:45 at RPE 2–3 10:00 at RPE 2–3 *Stretch Intervals*	**Foundation Run** 5:00 at RPE 2–3 30:00 at RPE 3–4	**Long Run with Fast Finish** 1 km at RPE 2–3 11 km at RPE 3–4 1 km at RPE 4–5
VO₂max Intervals 5:00 at RPE 2–3 5:00 at RPE 3–4 5 × 2:00 at RPE 7–8* / 2:00 at RPE 2–3 10:00 at RPE 2–3 *Precision Splitting*	**Foundation Run** 5:00 at RPE 2–3 35:00 at RPE 3–4	**Long Run with Fast Finish** 1 km at RPE 2–3 19 km at RPE 3–4 1 km at RPE 4–5
5K Pace Intervals 1 km at RPE 2–3 1 km at RPE 3–4 6 × (0.8 km at 5KP* / 1:00 rest) 2 km at RPE 2–3 *Precision Splitting*	**Foundation Run** 5:00 at RPE 2–3 40:00 at RPE 3–4	**Long Run with Fast Finish** 1 km at RPE 2–3 21 km at RPE 3–4 1 km at RPE 4–5
Hill Repetitions 5:00 at RPE 2–3 5:00 at RPE 3–4 8 × 1:00 uphill at RPE 8–9* / 2:00 at RPE 2–3 10:00 at RPE 2–3 *Stretch Intervals*	**Foundation Run** 5:00 at RPE 2–3 35:00 at RPE 3–4	**Long Run with Fast Finish** 1 km at RPE 2–3 13 km at RPE 3–4 1 km at RPE 4–5
The Prefontaine 1 km at RPE 2–3 1 km at RPE 3–4 ? × 200m at RPE 9 / 200m at RPE 6 1 km at RPE 2–3 1 km at RPE 3–4 *(? = Go to failure)*	**Foundation Run** 5:00 at RPE 2–3 40:00 at RPE 3–4	**Long Run with Fast Finish** 1 km at RPE 2–3 23 km at RPE 3–4 1 km at RPE 4–5
VO₂max Intervals 5:00 at RPE 2–3 5:00 at RPE 3–4 6 × 2:00 at RPE 7–8* / 2:00 at RPE 2–3 10:00 at RPE 2–3 *Precision Splitting*	**Foundation Run** 5:00 at RPE 2–3 45:00 at RPE 3–4	**Long Run with Fast Finish** 1 km at RPE 2–3 25 km at RPE 3–4 1 km at RPE 4–5

1 Marathon

	MONDAY	TUESDAY	WEDNESDAY	THURSDAY
12	Rest	**Fartleks** 5:00 at RPE 2–3 5:00 at RPE 3–4 1:00 at CV, 1:00 at RPE 2–3 2:00 at LTP, 1:00 at RPE 2–3 3:00 at SSP, 1:00 at RPE 2–3 2:00 at LTP, 1:00 at RPE 2–3 1:00 at CV, 1:00 at RPE 2–3 2:00 at LTP, 1:00 at RPE 2–3 1:00 at CV, 1:00 at RPE 2–3 2:00 at LTP, 1:00 at RPE 2–3 3:00 at SSP, 1:00 at RPE 2–3 10:00 at RPE 3–4	**Foundation Run** 5:00 at RPE 2–3 40:00 at RPE 3–4	**Foundation Run** 5:00 at RPE 2–3 40:00 at RPE 3–4
13	Rest	**Steady-State Run** 5:00 at RPE 2–3 5:00 at RPE 3–4 45:00 at RPE 5 10:00 at RPE 2–3	**Foundation Run** 5:00 at RPE 2–3 45:00 at RPE 3–4	**Foundation Run** 5:00 at RPE 2–3 45:00 at RPE 3–4
14	Rest	**Tempo Run** 5:00 at RPE 2–3 5:00 at RPE 3–4 14:00 at RPE 6 5:00 at RPE 2–3 14:00 at RPE 6 10:00 at RPE 2–3	**Foundation Run** 5:00 at RPE 2–3 50:00 at RPE 3–4	**Foundation Run** 5:00 at RPE 2–3 50:00 at RPE 3–4
15	Rest	**Progression Run** 5:00 at RPE 2–3 15:00 at RPE 3–4 12:00 at SSP 6:00 at LTP 3:00 at CV 5:00 at RPE 2–3	**Foundation Run** 5:00 at RPE 2–3 40:00 at RPE 3–4	**Foundation Run** 5:00 at RPE 2–3 40:00 at RPE 3–4
16	Rest	**Steady-State Run** 5:00 at RPE 2–3 5:00 at RPE 3–4 50:00 at RPE 5 10:00 at RPE 2–3	**Foundation Run** 5:00 at RPE 2–3 50:00 at RPE 3–4	**Foundation Run** 5:00 at RPE 2–3 50:00 at RPE 3–4
17	Rest	**Relaxed 10K Time Trial** 1 km at RPE 2–3 1 km at RPE 3–4 10 km at 95% effort 2 km at RPE 2–3	**Foundation Run** 5:00 at RPE 2–3 40:00 at RPE 3–4	**Foundation Run** 5:00 at RPE 2–3 40:00 at RPE 3–4
18	Rest	**Fartleks** 5:00 at RPE 2–3 5:00 at RPE 3–4 6 × 1:00 at RPE 7–8 / 2:00 at RPE 2–3 10:00 at RPE 3–4	**Foundation Run** 5:00 at RPE 2–3 40:00 at RPE 3–4	**Foundation Run** 5:00 at RPE 2–3 35:00 at RPE 3–4

How to Run the Perfect Race

FRIDAY	SATURDAY	SUNDAY
Speed Intervals 5:00 at RPE 2–3 5:00 at RPE 3–4 10 × 0:45 at RPE 8–9* / 1:45 at RPE 2–3 10:00 at RPE 2–3 *Stretch Intervals*	**Foundation Run** 5:00 at RPE 2–3 40:00 at RPE 3–4	**Long Run with Fast Finish** 1 km at RPE 2–3 15 km at RPE 3–4 1 km at RPE 4–5
5K Pace Intervals 1 km at RPE 2–3 1 km at RPE 3–4 8 × (0.6 km at 5KP* / 1:00 rest) 2 km at RPE 2–3 *Precision Splitting*	**Foundation Run** 5:00 at RPE 2–3 45:00 at RPE 3–4	**Long Run with Fast Finish** 1 km at RPE 2–3 27 km at RPE 3–4 1 km at RPE 4–5
Relaxed 5K Time Trial 1 km at RPE 2–3 1 km at RPE 3–4 5 km at 95% effort 2 km at RPE 2–3	**Foundation Run** 5:00 at RPE 2–3 50:00 at RPE 3–4	**Long Run with Fast Finish** 1 km at RPE 2–3 29 km at RPE 3–4 1 km at RPE 4–5
Hill Repetitions 5:00 at RPE 2–3 5:00 at RPE 3–4 4 × 2:00 uphill at RPE 7–8* / 2:00 at RPE 2–3 10:00 at RPE 2–3 *Stretch Intervals*	**Foundation Run** 5:00 at RPE 2–3 40:00 at RPE 3–4	**Long Run with Fast Finish** 1 km at RPE 2–3 17 km at RPE 3–4 1 km at RPE 4–5
Speed Intervals 5:00 at RPE 2–3 5:00 at RPE 3–4 8 × 1:00 at RPE 8–9* / 2:00 at RPE 2–3 10:00 at RPE 2–3 *Stretch Intervals*	**Foundation Run** 5:00 at RPE 2–3 50:00 at RPE 3–4	**Marathon Pace Run** 1 km (0.6 mile) at RPE 2–3 2 km (1.2 miles) at RPE 3–4 20 km (12.4 miles) at MP 2 km (1.2 miles) at RPE 2–3
VO$_2$max Intervals 5:00 at RPE 2–3 5:00 at RPE 3–4 5 × 2:00 at RPE 7–8* / 2:00 at RPE 2–3 10:00 at RPE 2–3 *Precision Splitting*	**Foundation Run** 5:00 at RPE 2–3 40:00 at RPE 3–4	**Long Run with Fast Finish** 1 km at RPE 2–3 15 km at RPE 3–4 1 km at RPE 4–5
Fast Finish Run 5:00 at RPE 2–3 15:00 at RPE 3–4 10:00 at RPE 6	**Foundation Run** 5:00 at RPE 2–3 15:00 at RPE 3–4	**Marathon Race**

Marathon

1

Marathon

This plan is a good fit for experienced competitive runners who are prepared to train hard in pursuit of improved marathon performance. Before starting the plan, be sure to build your training to the point where you're comfortably able to run 7 days a week for up to 17 km.

	MONDAY	TUESDAY	WEDNESDAY	THURSDAY
1	**Recovery Run** 30:00 at RPE 2–3	**Progression Run** 5:00 at RPE 2–3 25:00 at RPE 3–4 8:00 at SSP 4:00 at LTP 2:00 at CV 5:00 at RPE 2–3	**Foundation Run** 5:00 at RPE 2–3 40:00 at RPE 3–4	**Foundation Run** 5:00 at RPE 2–3 40:00 at RPE 3–4
2	**Recovery Run** 30:00 at RPE 2–3	**Progression Run** 5:00 at RPE 2–3 35:00 at RPE 3–4 4:00 at LTP 2:00 at CV 1:00 at MAS 5:00 at RPE 2–3	**Foundation Run** 5:00 at RPE 2–3 45:00 at RPE 3–4	**Foundation Run** 5:00 at RPE 2–3 45:00 at RPE 3–4
3	Rest	**Progression Run** 5:00 at RPE 2–3 25:00 at RPE 3–4 8:00 at SSP 4:00 at LTP 2:00 at CV 5:00 at RPE 2–3	**Foundation Run** 5:00 at RPE 2–3 40:00 at RPE 3–4	**Foundation Run** 5:00 at RPE 2–3 40:00 at RPE 3–4
4	**Recovery Run** 30:00 at RPE 2–3	**Mini Intervals** 5:00 at RPE 2–3 10:00 at RPE 3–4 40 × (0:30 at 10KP / 0:30 at RPE 2–3) 15:00 at RPE 2–3	**Foundation Run** 5:00 at RPE 2–3 45:00 at RPE 3–4	**Foundation Run** 5:00 at RPE 2–3 45:00 at RPE 3–4
5	**Recovery Run** 30:00 at RPE 2–3	**Critical Velocity Intervals** 5:00 at RPE 2–3 10:00 at RPE 3–4 6 × 4:00 at RPE 6–7* / 2:00 at RPE 2–3 15:00 at RPE 2–3 *Precision Splitting*	**Foundation Run** 5:00 at RPE 2–3 50:00 at RPE 3–4	**Foundation Run** 5:00 at RPE 2–3 50:00 at RPE 3–4

LEVEL

SSP Steady-State Pace
LTP Lactate Threshold Pace
CV Critical Velocity
MAS Maximal Aerobic Speed

5KP 5K Pace
10KP 10K Pace
MP Marathon Pace

FRIDAY	SATURDAY	SUNDAY
Fartleks 5:00 at RPE 2–3 10:00 at RPE 3–4 8 × 1:00 at RPE 7–8 / 2:00 at RPE 2–3 15:00 at RPE 3–4	**Foundation Run** 5:00 at RPE 2–3 40:00 at RPE 3–4	**Long Run with Fast Finish** 1 km at RPE 2–3 15 km at RPE 3–4 1 km at RPE 4–5
Fartleks 5:00 at RPE 2–3 10:00 at RPE 3–4 8 × 0:20 at RPE 8–9 / 1:40 at RPE 2–3 15:00 at RPE 3–4	**Foundation Run** 5:00 at RPE 2–3 45:00 at RPE 3–4	**Long Run with Fast Finish** 1 km at RPE 2–3 17 km at RPE 3–4 1 km at RPE 4–5
Fartleks 5:00 at RPE 2–3 10:00 at RPE 3–4 8 × 1:00 at RPE 7–8 / 2:00 at RPE 2–3 15:00 at RPE 3–4	**Foundation Run** 5:00 at RPE 2–3 40:00 at RPE 3–4	**Long Run with Fast Finish** 1 km at RPE 2–3 15 km at RPE 3–4 1 km at RPE 4–5
Hill Repetitions 5:00 at RPE 2–3 10:00 at RPE 3–4 10 × 0:30 uphill at RPE 8–9* / 1:30 at RPE 2–3 15:00 at RPE 2–3 *Stretch Intervals*	**Foundation Run** 5:00 at RPE 2–3 45:00 at RPE 3–4	**Long Run with Fast Finish** 1 km at RPE 2–3 21 km at RPE 3–4 1 km at RPE 4–5
Accelerations 5:00 at RPE 2–3 10:00 at RPE 3–4 11:00 acceleration 10:00 at RPE 2–3 6:00 acceleration 10:00 at RPE 2–3	**Foundation Run** 5:00 at RPE 2–3 50:00 at RPE 3–4	**Long Run with Fast Finish** 1 km at RPE 2–3 25 km at RPE 3–4 1 km at RPE 4–5

2 Marathon

	MONDAY	TUESDAY	WEDNESDAY	THURSDAY
6	Rest	**Fartleks** 5:00 at RPE 2–3 10:00 at RPE 3–4 1:00 at CV, 1:00 at RPE 2–3 2:00 at LTP, 1:00 at RPE 2–3 3:00 at SSP, 1:00 at RPE 2–3 2:00 at LTP, 1:00 at RPE 2–3 1:00 at CV, 1:00 at RPE 2–3 2:00 at LTP, 1:00 at RPE 2–3 3:00 at SSP, 1:00 at RPE 2–3 15:00 at RPE 3–4	**Foundation Run** 5:00 at RPE 2–3 45:00 at RPE 3–4	**Foundation Run** 5:00 at RPE 2–3 45:00 at RPE 3–4
7	**Recovery Run** 30:00 at RPE 2–3	**Steady-State Run** 5:00 at RPE 2–3 10:00 at RPE 3–4 45:00 at RPE 5 15:00 at RPE 2–3	**Foundation Run** 5:00 at RPE 2–3 50:00 at RPE 3–4	**Foundation Run** 5:00 at RPE 2–3 50:00 at RPE 3–4
8	**Recovery Run** 30:00 at RPE 2–3	**Tempo Run** 5:00 at RPE 2–3 10:00 at RPE 3–4 16:00 at RPE 6 5:00 at RPE 2–3 16:00 at RPE 6 15:00 at RPE 2–3	**Foundation Run** 5:00 at RPE 2–3 55:00 at RPE 3–4	**Foundation Run** 5:00 at RPE 2–3 55:00 at RPE 3–4
9	Rest	**Progression Run** 5:00 at RPE 2–3 35:00 at RPE 3–4 8:00 at LTP 4:00 at CV 2:00 at MAS 5:00 at RPE 2–3	**Foundation Run** 5:00 at RPE 2–3 45:00 at RPE 3–4	**Foundation Run** 5:00 at RPE 2–3 45:00 at RPE 3–4
10	**Recovery Run** 30:00 at RPE 2–3	**Mini Intervals** 5:00 at RPE 2–3 10:00 at RPE 3–4 30 × (0:30 at CV / 0:30 at RPE 2–3) 15:00 at RPE 2–3	**Foundation Run** 5:00 at RPE 2–3 55:00 at RPE 3–4	**Foundation Run** 5:00 at RPE 2–3 55:00 at RPE 3–4
11	**Recovery Run** 30:00 at RPE 2–3	**Critical Velocity Intervals** 5:00 at RPE 2–3 10:00 at RPE 3–4 7 × 4:00 at RPE 6–7* / 2:00 at RPE 2–3 15:00 at RPE 2–3 *Precision Splitting*	**Foundation Run** 5:00 at RPE 2–3 55:00 at RPE 3–4	**Foundation Run** 5:00 at RPE 2–3 55:00 at RPE 3–4

FRIDAY	SATURDAY	SUNDAY
Speed Intervals 5:00 at RPE 2–3 10:00 at RPE 3–4 10 × 0:45 at RPE 8–9* / 1:45 at RPE 2–3 15:00 at RPE 2–3 *Stretch Intervals*	**Foundation Run** 5:00 at RPE 2–3 45:00 at RPE 3–4	**Long Run with Fast Finish** 1 km at RPE 2–3 17 km at RPE 3–4 1 km at RPE 4–5
VO$_2$max Intervals 5:00 at RPE 2–3 10:00 at RPE 3–4 6 × 2:00 at RPE 7–8* / 2:00 at RPE 2–3 15:00 at RPE 2–3 *Precision Splitting*	**Foundation Run** 5:00 at RPE 2–3 50:00 at RPE 3–4	**Depletion Run** 5:00 at RPE 2–3 1:55:00 at RPE 3–4 *No calories before or during*
5K Pace Intervals 1 km at RPE 2–3 2.5 km at RPE 3–4 6 × (0.8 km at 5KP* / 1:00 rest) 3.5 km at RPE 2–3 *Precision Splitting*	**Foundation Run** 5:00 at RPE 2–3 55:00 at RPE 3–4	**Marathon Pace Run** 1 km (0.6 mile) at RPE 2–3 2 km (1.2 miles) at RPE 3–4 6 × 1.5 km (0.9 mile) at MP / 1.5 km (0.9 mile) at RPE 3–4 2 km (1.2 miles) at RPE 2–3
Hill Repetitions 5:00 at RPE 2–3 10:00 at RPE 3–4 8 × 1:00 uphill at RPE 8–9* / 2:00 at RPE 2–3 15:00 at RPE 2–3 *Stretch Intervals*	**Foundation Run** 5:00 at RPE 2–3 45:00 at RPE 3–4	**Long Run with Fast Finish** 1 km at RPE 2–3 19 km at RPE 3–4 1 km at RPE 4–5
The Prefontaine 1 km at RPE 2–3 2.5 km at RPE 3–4 ? × 200m at RPE 9 / 200m at RPE 6 1 km at RPE 2–3 2.5 km at RPE 3–4 *(? = Go to failure)*	**Foundation Run** 5:00 at RPE 2–3 55:00 at RPE 3–4	**Long Run with Fast Finish** 1 km at RPE 2–3 29 km at RPE 3–4 1 km at RPE 4–5
VO$_2$max Intervals 5:00 at RPE 2–3 10:00 at RPE 3–4 7 × 2:00 at RPE 7–8* / 2:00 at RPE 2–3 15:00 at RPE 2–3 *Precision Splitting*	**Foundation Run** 5:00 at RPE 2–3 55:00 at RPE 3–4	**Marathon Pace Run** 1 km (0.6 mile) at RPE 2–3 2 km (1.2 miles) at RPE 3–4 20 km (12.4 miles) at MP 2 km (1.2 miles) at RPE 2–3

2 Marathon

	MONDAY	TUESDAY	WEDNESDAY	THURSDAY
12	Rest	**Fartleks** 5:00 at RPE 2–3 10:00 at RPE 3–4 1:00 at CV, 1:00 at RPE 2–3 2:00 at LTP, 1:00 at RPE 2–3 3:00 at SSP, 1:00 at RPE 2–3 2:00 at LTP, 1:00 at RPE 2–3 1:00 at CV, 1:00 at RPE 2–3 2:00 at LTP, 1:00 at RPE 2–3 3:00 at SSP, 1:00 at RPE 2–3 2:00 at LTP, 1:00 at RPE 2–3 1:00 at CV, 1:00 at RPE 2–3 15:00 at RPE 3–4	**Foundation Run** 5:00 at RPE 2–3 50:00 at RPE 3–4	**Foundation Run** 5:00 at RPE 2–3 50:00 at RPE 3–4
13	**Recovery Run** 30:00 at RPE 2–3	**Steady-State Run** 5:00 at RPE 2–3 10:00 at RPE 3–4 50:00 at RPE 5 15:00 at RPE 2–3	**Foundation Run** 5:00 at RPE 2–3 55:00 at RPE 3–4	**Foundation Run** 5:00 at RPE 2–3 55:00 at RPE 3–4
14	**Recovery Run** 30:00 at RPE 2–3	**Tempo Run** 5:00 at RPE 2–3 10:00 at RPE 3–4 20:00 at RPE 6 5:00 at RPE 2–3 20:00 at RPE 6 15:00 at RPE 2–3	**Foundation Run** 5:00 at RPE 2–3 55:00 at RPE 3–4	**Foundation Run** 5:00 at RPE 2–3 55:00 at RPE 3–4
15	Rest	**Progression Run** 5:00 at RPE 2–3 25:00 at RPE 3–4 12:00 at SSP 6:00 at LTP 3:00 at CV 5:00 at RPE 2–3	**Foundation Run** 5:00 at RPE 2–3 50:00 at RPE 3–4	**Foundation Run** 5:00 at RPE 2–3 50:00 at RPE 3–4
16	**Recovery Run** 30:00 at RPE 2–3	**Steady-State Run** 5:00 at RPE 2–3 10:00 at RPE 3–4 55:00 at RPE 5 15:00 at RPE 2–3	**Foundation Run** 5:00 at RPE 2–3 55:00 at RPE 3–4	**Foundation Run** 5:00 at RPE 2–3 55:00 at RPE 3–4
17	**Recovery Run** 30:00 at RPE 2–3	**Relaxed 10K Time Trial** 1 km at RPE 2–3 2.5 km at RPE 3–4 10 km at 95% effort 3.5 km at RPE 2–3	**Foundation Run** 5:00 at RPE 2–3 55:00 at RPE 3–4	**Foundation Run** 5:00 at RPE 2–3 50:00 at RPE 3–4
18	Rest	**Fartleks** 5:00 at RPE 2–3 10:00 at RPE 3–4 8 × 1:00 at RPE 7–8 / 2:00 at RPE 2–3 15:00 at RPE 3–4	**Foundation Run** 5:00 at RPE 2–3 40:00 at RPE 3–4	**Foundation Run** 5:00 at RPE 2–3 35:00 at RPE 3–4

How to Run the Perfect Race

FRIDAY	SATURDAY	SUNDAY
Speed Intervals 5:00 at RPE 2–3 10:00 at RPE 3–4 10 × 0:45 at RPE 8–9* / 1:45 at RPE 2–3 15:00 at RPE 2–3 *Stretch Intervals	**Foundation Run** 5:00 at RPE 2–3 50:00 at RPE 3–4	**Depletion Run** 5:00 at RPE 2–3 2:15:00 at RPE 3–4 *No calories before or during*
5K Pace Intervals 1 km at RPE 2–3 2.5 km at RPE 3–4 8 × (0.6 km at 5KP* / 1:00 rest) 3.5 km at RPE 2–3 *Precision Splitting	**Foundation Run** 5:00 at RPE 2–3 55:00 at RPE 3–4	**Long Run with Fast Finish** 1 km at RPE 2–3 30 km at RPE 3–4 2 km at RPE 5–6* *Note the slightly more aggressive fast finish.*
Relaxed 5K Time Trial 1 km at RPE 2–3 2.5 km at RPE 3–4 5 km at 95% effort 3.5 km at RPE 2–3	**Foundation Run** 5:00 at RPE 2–3 55:00 at RPE 3–4	**Long Run with Fast Finish** 1 km at RPE 2–3 32 km at RPE 3–4 2 km at RPE 5–6* *Note the slightly more aggressive fast finish.*
Hill Repetitions 5:00 at RPE 2–3 10:00 at RPE 3–4 5 × 2:00 uphill at RPE 7–8* / 2:00 at RPE 2–3 15:00 at RPE 2–3 *Stretch Intervals	**Foundation Run** 5:00 at RPE 2–3 50:00 at RPE 3–4	**Depletion Run** 5:00 at RPE 2–3 2:35:00 at RPE 3–4 *No calories before or during*
Speed Intervals 5:00 at RPE 2–3 10:00 at RPE 3–4 8 × 1:00 at RPE 8–9* / 2:00 at RPE 2–3 15:00 at RPE 2–3 *Stretch Intervals	**Foundation Run** 5:00 at RPE 2–3 55:00 at RPE 3–4	**Marathon Pace Run** 1 km (0.6 mile) at RPE 2–3 2 km (1.2 miles) at RPE 3–4 26 km (16.1 miles) at MP 2 km (1.2 miles) at RPE 2–3
VO$_2$max Intervals 5:00 at RPE 2–3 10:00 at RPE 3–4 6 × 2:00 at RPE 7–8* / 2:00 at RPE 2–3 15:00 at RPE 2–3 *Precision Splitting	**Foundation Run** 5:00 at RPE 2–3 45:00 at RPE 3–4	**Long Run with Fast Finish** 1 km at RPE 2–3 16 km at RPE 3–4 2 km at RPE 5–6* *Note the slightly more aggressive fast finish.*
Fast Finish Run 5:00 at RPE 2–3 20:00 at RPE 3–4 10:00 at RPE 6	**Foundation Run** 5:00 at RPE 2–3 15:00 at RPE 3–4	**Marathon Race**

2 Marathon

Marathon

This plan is designed for runners seeking the absolute limit of their potential at the marathon distance. Before starting the plan, be sure to build your training to the point where you're comfortably able to run 9 times per week for up to 23 km.

	MONDAY	TUESDAY	WEDNESDAY	THURSDAY
1	**Recovery Run** 40:00 at RPE 2–3	**Progression Run** 5:00 at RPE 2–3 35:00 at RPE 3–4 8:00 at SSP 4:00 at LTP 2:00 at CV 5:00 at RPE 2–3 **Recovery Run** 20:00 at RPE 2–3	**Foundation Run** 5:00 at RPE 2–3 55:00 at RPE 3–4	**Foundation Run** 5:00 at RPE 2–3 55:00 at RPE 3–4
2	**Recovery Run** 40:00 at RPE 2–3	**Progression Run** 5:00 at RPE 2–3 40:00 at RPE 3–4 4:00 at LTP 2:00 at CV 1:00 at MAS 5:00 at RPE 2–3 **Recovery Run** 20:00 at RPE 2–3	**Foundation Run** 5:00 at RPE 2–3 55:00 at RPE 3–4	**Foundation Run** 5:00 at RPE 2–3 55:00 at RPE 3–4
3	Rest	**Progression Run** 5:00 at RPE 2–3 35:00 at RPE 3–4 8:00 at SSP 4:00 at LTP 2:00 at CV 5:00 at RPE 2–3 **Recovery Run** 20:00 at RPE 2–3	**Foundation Run** 5:00 at RPE 2–3 55:00 at RPE 3–4	**Foundation Run** 5:00 at RPE 2–3 55:00 at RPE 3–4

LEVEL

SSP Steady-State Pace
LTP Lactate Threshold Pace
CV Critical Velocity
MAS Maximal Aerobic Speed

5KP 5K Pace
10KP 10K Pace
HMP Half-Marathon Pace
MP Marathon Pace

FRIDAY	SATURDAY	SUNDAY
Fartleks 5:00 at RPE 2–3 10:00 at RPE 3–4 8 × 1:00 at RPE 7–8 / 2:00 at RPE 2–3 15:00 at RPE 3–4 **Recovery Run** 20:00 at RPE 2–3	**Foundation Run** 5:00 at RPE 2–3 55:00 at RPE 3–4	**Long Run with Fast Finish** 1 km at RPE 2–3 21 km at RPE 3–4 1 km at RPE 4–5
Fartleks 5:00 at RPE 2–3 15:00 at RPE 3–4 10 × 0:20 at RPE 8–9 / 1:40 at RPE 2–3 20:00 at RPE 3–4 **Recovery Run** 20:00 at RPE 2–3	**Foundation Run** 5:00 at RPE 2–3 55:00 at RPE 3–4	**Long Run with Fast Finish** 1 km at RPE 2–3 25 km at RPE 3–4 1 km at RPE 4–5
Fartleks 5:00 at RPE 2–3 10:00 at RPE 3–4 8 × 1:00 at RPE 7–8 / 2:00 at RPE 2–3 15:00 at RPE 3–4 **Recovery Run** 20:00 at RPE 2–3	**Foundation Run** 5:00 at RPE 2–3 55:00 at RPE 3–4	**Depletion Run** 5:00 at RPE 2–3 1:35:00 at RPE 3–4 *No calories before or during*

3 Marathon

	MONDAY	TUESDAY	WEDNESDAY	THURSDAY
4	**Recovery Run** 40:00 at RPE 2–3	**Mini Intervals** 5:00 at RPE 2–3 15:00 at RPE 3–4 50 × (0:30 at 10KP / 0:30 at RPE 2–3) 20:00 at RPE 2–3 **Recovery Run** 25:00 at RPE 2–3	**Foundation Run** 5:00 at RPE 2–3 55:00 at RPE 3–4	**Foundation Run** 5:00 at RPE 2–3 1:00:00 at RPE 3–4
5	**Recovery Run** 40:00 at RPE 2–3	**Critical Velocity Intervals** 5:00 at RPE 2–3 15:00 at RPE 3–4 7 × 4:00* at RPE 6–7 / 2:00 at RPE 2–3 20:00 at RPE 2–3 *Precision Splitting* **Recovery Run** 25:00 at RPE 2–3	**Foundation Run** 5:00 at RPE 2–3 55:00 at RPE 3–4	**Foundation Run** 5:00 at RPE 2–3 1:00:00 at RPE 3–4
6	Rest	**Fartleks** 5:00 at RPE 2–3 15:00 at RPE 3–4 1:00 at CV, 1:00 at RPE 2–3 2:00 at LTP, 1:00 at RPE 2–3 3:00 at SSP, 1:00 at RPE 2–3 2:00 at LTP, 1:00 at RPE 2–3 1:00 at CV, 1:00 at RPE 2–3 2:00 at LTP, 1:00 at RPE 2–3 3:00 at SSP, 1:00 at RPE 2–3 2:00 at LTP, 1:00 at RPE 2–3 1:00 at CV, 1:00 at RPE 2–3 20:00 at RPE 3–4 **Recovery Run** 20:00 at RPE 2–3	**Foundation Run** 5:00 at RPE 2–3 55:00 at RPE 3–4	**Foundation Run** 5:00 at RPE 2–3 55:00 at RPE 3–4
7	**Recovery Run** 40:00 at RPE 2–3	**Steady-State Run** 5:00 at RPE 2–3 15:00 at RPE 3–4 50:00 at RPE 5 20:00 at RPE 2–3 **Recovery Run** 30:00 at RPE 2–3	**Foundation Run** 5:00 at RPE 2–3 55:00 at RPE 3–4	**Foundation Run** 5:00 at RPE 2–3 1:05:00 at RPE 3–4
8	**Recovery Run** 40:00 at RPE 2–3	**Tempo Run** 5:00 at RPE 2–3 15:00 at RPE 3–4 18:00 at RPE 6 5:00 at RPE 2–3 18:00 at RPE 6 20:00 at RPE 2–3 **Recovery Run** 30:00 at RPE 2–3	**Foundation Run** 5:00 at RPE 2–3 55:00 at RPE 3–4	**Foundation Run** 5:00 at RPE 2–3 1:05:00 at RPE 3–4

How to Run the Perfect Race

FRIDAY	SATURDAY	SUNDAY
Hill Repetitions 5:00 at RPE 2–3 15.00 at RPE 3–4 12 × 0:30 uphill at RPE 8–9 / 1:30 at RPE 2–3 20:00 at RPE 2–3 *Precision Splitting* **Recovery Run** 25:00 at RPE 2–3	**Foundation Run** 5:00 at RPE 2–3 55:00 at RPE 3–4	**Half-Marathon Pace Run** 1 km at RPE 2–3 4 km at RPE 3–4 3 × (3 km at HMP / 1:00 rest) 5 km at RPE 2–3
Accelerations 5:00 at RPE 2–3 15:00 at RPE 3–4 11:00 acceleration 10:00 at RPE 2–3 6:00 acceleration 10:00 at RPE 2–3 11:00 acceleration 20:00 at RPE 2–3 **Recovery Run** 25:00 at RPE 2–3	**Foundation Run** 5:00 at RPE 2–3 55:00 at RPE 3–4	**Long Run with Fast Finish** 1 km at RPE 2–3 27 km at RPE 3–4 1 km at RPE 4–5
Speed Intervals 5:00 at RPE 2–3 15:00 at RPE 3–4 12 × 0:45* at RPE 8–9 / 1:45 at RPE 2–3 20:00 at RPE 2–3 *Stretch Intervals* **Recovery Run** 20:00 at RPE 2–3	**Foundation Run** 5:00 at RPE 2–3 55:00 at RPE 3–4	**Depletion Run** 5:00 at RPE 2–3 1:55:00 at RPE 3–4 *No calories before or during*
VO$_2$max Intervals 5:00 at RPE 2–3 15:00 at RPE 3–4 7 × 2:00* at RPE 7–8 / 1:00 at RPE 2–3 20:00 at RPE 2–3 *Precision Splitting* **Recovery Run** 30:00 at RPE 2–3	**Foundation Run** 5:00 at RPE 2–3 55:00 at RPE 3–4	**Long Run with Fast Finish** 1 km at RPE 2–3 30 km at RPE 3–4 2 km at RPE 5–6* *Note the slightly more aggressive fast finish.*
5K Pace Intervals 1 km at RPE 2–3 4 km at RPE 3–4 6 × (0.8 km at 5KP* / 1:00 rest) 5 km at RPE 2–3 *Precision Splitting* **Recovery Run** 30:00 at RPE 2–3	**Foundation Run** 5:00 at RPE 2–3 55:00 at RPE 3–4	**Marathon Pace Run** 1 km (0.6 mile) at RPE 2–3 2 km (1.2 miles) at RPE 3–4 6 × 1.5 km (0.9 mile) at MP / 1.5 km (0.9 mile) at RPE 3–4 2 km (1.2 miles) at RPE 2–3

3 Marathon

	MONDAY	TUESDAY	WEDNESDAY	THURSDAY
9	Rest	**Progression Run** 5:00 at RPE 2–3 40:00 at RPE 3–4 4:00 at LTP 2:00 at CV 1:00 at MAS 5:00 at RPE 2–3 **Recovery Run** 25:00 at RPE 2–3	**Foundation Run** 5:00 at RPE 2–3 55:00 at RPE 3–4	**Foundation Run** 5:00 at RPE 2–3 55:00 at RPE 3–4
10	**Recovery Run** 40:00 at RPE 2–3	**Mini Intervals** 5:00 at RPE 2–3 15:00 at RPE 3–4 50 × (0:30 at CV / 0:30 at RPE 2–3) 20:00 at RPE 2–3 **Recovery Run** 35:00 at RPE 2–3	**Foundation Run** 5:00 at RPE 2–3 55:00 at RPE 3–4	**Foundation Run** 5:00 at RPE 2–3 1:10:00 at RPE 3–4
11	**Recovery Run** 40:00 at RPE 2–3	**Critical Velocity Intervals** 5:00 at RPE 2–3 15:00 at RPE 3–4 8 × 4:00* at RPE 6–7 / 2:00 at RPE 2–3 20:00 at RPE 2–3 *Precision Splitting* **Recovery Run** 35:00 at RPE 2–3	**Foundation Run** 5:00 at RPE 2–3 55:00 at RPE 3–4	**Foundation Run** 5:00 at RPE 2–3 1:10:00 at RPE 3–4
12	Rest	**Fartleks** 5:00 at RPE 2–3 15:00 at RPE 3–4 1:00 at CV, 1:00 at RPE 2–3 2:00 at LTP, 1:00 at RPE 2–3 3:00 at SSP, 1:00 at RPE 2–3 2:00 at LTP, 1:00 at RPE 2–3 1:00 at CV, 1:00 at RPE 2–3 2:00 at LTP, 1:00 at RPE 2–3 3:00 at SSP, 1:00 at RPE 2–3 2:00 at LTP, 1:00 at RPE 2–3 1:00 at CV, 1:00 at RPE 2–3 20:00 at RPE 3–4 **Recovery Run** 30:00 at RPE 2–3	**Foundation Run** 5:00 at RPE 2–3 55:00 at RPE 3–4	**Foundation Run** 5:00 at RPE 2–3 55:00 at RPE 3–4
13	**Recovery Run** 40:00 at RPE 2–3	**Steady-State Run** 5:00 at RPE 2–3 15:00 at RPE 3–4 1:00:00 at RPE 5 20:00 at RPE 2–3 **Recovery Run** 40:00 at RPE 2–3	**Foundation Run** 5:00 at RPE 2–3 55:00 at RPE 3–4	**Foundation Run** 5:00 at RPE 2–3 1:10:00 at RPE 3–4

How to Run the Perfect Race

FRIDAY	SATURDAY	SUNDAY
Hill Repetitions 5:00 at RPE 2–3 15:00 at RPE 3–4 10 × 1:00 uphill at RPE 8–9* / 2:00 at RPE 2–3 20:00 at RPE 2–3 *Stretch Intervals **Recovery Run** 25:00 at RPE 2–3	**Foundation Run** 5:00 at RPE 2–3 55:00 at RPE 3–4	**Long Run with Fast Finish** 1 km at RPE 2–3 19 km at RPE 3–4 1 km at RPE 4–5
The Prefontaine 1 km at RPE 2–3 4 km at RPE 3–4 ? × 200m at RPE 9 / 200m at RPE 6 1 km at RPE 2–3 4 km at RPE 3–4 (? = Go to failure) **Recovery Run** 35:00 at RPE 2–3	**Foundation Run** 5:00 at RPE 2–3 55:00 at RPE 3–4	**Long Run with Fast Finish** 1 km at RPE 2–3 30 km at RPE 3–4 2 km at RPE 5–6* *Note the slightly more aggressive fast finish.
Fartleks 5:00 at RPE 2–3 15:00 at RPE 3–4 10 × 0:20 at RPE 8–9 / 1:40 at RPE 2–3 20:00 at RPE 3–4 **Recovery Run** 35:00 at RPE 2–3	**Foundation Run** 5:00 at RPE 2–3 55:00 at RPE 3–4	**Marathon Pace Run** 1 km (0.6 mile) at RPE 2–3 2 km (1.2 miles) at RPE 3–4 20 km (12.4 miles) at MP 2 km (1.2 miles) at RPE 2–3
VO$_2$max Intervals 5:00 at RPE 2–3 15:00 at RPE 3–4 6 × 2:00 at RPE 7–8* / 1:00 at RPE 2–3 20:00 at RPE 2–3 *Precision Splitting **Recovery Run** 30:00 at RPE 2–3	**Foundation Run** 5:00 at RPE 2–3 55:00 at RPE 3–4	**Depletion Run** 5:00 at RPE 2–3 2:15:00 at RPE 3–4 No calories before or during
5K Pace Intervals 1 km at RPE 2–3 4 km at RPE 3–4 8 × (0.6 km at 5KP* / 1:00 rest) 5 km at RPE 2–3 *Precision Splitting **Recovery Run** 40:00 at RPE 2–3	**Foundation Run** 5:00 at RPE 2–3 55:00 at RPE 3–4	**Marathon Pace Run** 1 km at RPE 2–3 15 km at RPE 3–4 16 km at MP

3 Marathon

	MONDAY	TUESDAY	WEDNESDAY	THURSDAY
14	**Recovery Run** 40:00 at RPE 2–3	**Tempo Run** 5:00 at RPE 2–3 15:00 at RPE 3–4 22:00 at RPE 6 5:00 at RPE 2–3 22:00 at RPE 6 20:00 at RPE 2–3 **Recovery Run** 40:00 at RPE 2–3	**Foundation Run** 5:00 at RPE 2–3 55:00 at RPE 3–4	**Foundation Run** 5:00 at RPE 2–3 1:10:00 at RPE 3–4
15	Rest	**Progression Run** 5:00 at RPE 2–3 25:00 at RPE 3–4 16:00 at SSP 8:00 at LTP 4:00 at CV 5:00 at RPE 2–3 **Recovery Run** 30:00 at RPE 2–3	**Foundation Run** 5:00 at RPE 2–3 55:00 at RPE 3–4	**Foundation Run** 5:00 at RPE 2–3 55:00 at RPE 3–4
16	**Recovery Run** 40:00 at RPE 2–3	**Steady-State Run** 5:00 at RPE 2–3 15:00 at RPE 3–4 1:10:00 at RPE 5 20:00 at RPE 2–3 **Recovery Run** 40:00 at RPE 2–3	**Foundation Run** 5:00 at RPE 2–3 55:00 at RPE 3–4	**Foundation Run** 5:00 at RPE 2–3 1:10:00 at RPE 3–4
17	**Recovery Run** 40:00 at RPE 2–3	**Relaxed 10K Time Trial** 1 km at RPE 2–3 4 km at RPE 3–4 10 km at 95% effort 5 km at RPE 2–3 **Recovery Run** 30:00 at RPE 2–3	**Foundation Run** 5:00 at RPE 2–3 55:00 at RPE 3–4	**Foundation Run** 5:00 at RPE 2–3 55:00 at RPE 3–4
18	Rest	**Fartleks** 5:00 at RPE 2–3 15:00 at RPE 3–4 10 × 1:00 at RPE 7–8 / 2:00 at RPE 2–3 20:00 at RPE 3–4	**Foundation Run** 5:00 at RPE 2–3 40:00 at RPE 3–4	**Foundation Run** 5:00 at RPE 2–3 40:00 at RPE 3–4

How to Run the Perfect Race

FRIDAY	SATURDAY	SUNDAY
Relaxed 5K Time Trial 1 km at RPE 2–3 4 km at RPE 3–4 5 km at 95% effort 5 km at RPE 2–3 **Recovery Run** 40:00 at RPE 2–3	**Foundation Run** 5:00 at RPE 2–3 55:00 at RPE 3–4	**Long Run with Fast Finish** 1 km at RPE 2–3 32 km at RPE 3–4 2 km at RPE 5–6* *Note the slightly more aggressive fast finish.*
Hill Repetitions 5:00 at RPE 2–3 15:00 at RPE 3–4 6 × 2:00 at RPE 7–8* / 2:00 at RPE 2–3 20:00 at RPE 2–3 *Stretch Intervals* **Recovery Run** 30:00 at RPE 2–3	**Foundation Run** 5:00 at RPE 2–3 55:00 at RPE 3–4	**Depletion Run** 5:00 at RPE 2–3 2:35:00 at RPE 3–4 *No calories before or during*
Speed Intervals 5:00 at RPE 2–3 15:00 at RPE 3–4 10 × 1:00* at RPE 8–9 / 2:00 at RPE 2–3 20:00 at RPE 2–3 *Stretch Intervals* **Recovery Run** 40:00 at RPE 2–3	**Foundation Run** 5:00 at RPE 2–3 55:00 at RPE 3–4	**Marathon Pace Run** 1 km (0.6 mile) at RPE 2–3 2 km (1.2 miles) at RPE 3–4 26 km (16.1 miles) at MP 2 km (1.2 miles) at RPE 2–3
VO₂max Intervals 5:00 at RPE 2–3 15:00 at RPE 3–4 6 × 2:00 at RPE 7–8* / 1:00 at RPE 2–3 20:00 at RPE 2–3 *Precision Splitting* **Recovery Run** 30:00 at RPE 2–3	**Foundation Run** 5:00 at RPE 2–3 55:00 at RPE 3–4	**Long Run with Fast Finish** 1 km at RPE 2–3 16 km at RPE 3–4 2 km at RPE 5–6* *Note the slightly more aggressive fast finish.*
Fast Finish Run 5:00 at RPE 2–3 20:00 at RPE 3–4 10:00 at RPE 6	**Foundation Run** 5:00 at RPE 2–3 15:00 at RPE 3–4	**Marathon Race**

Marathon

REFERENCES

Albertus, Y., R. Tucker, A. St. Clair Gibson, E. V. Lambert, D. B. Hampson, and T. D. Noakes. "Effect of Distance Feedback on Pacing Strategy and Perceived Exertion during Cycling." *Medicine & Science in Sports & Exercise* 37, no. 3 (2005): 461–468.

Bassett, D. R., Jr. "Scientific Contributions of A. V. Hill: Exercise Physiology Pioneer." *Journal of Applied Physiology* 93, no. 5 (2002): 1567–1582. https://doi.org/10.1152/japplphysiol.01246.2001.

Blanchfield, Anthony William, James Hardy, Helma Majella De Morree, Walter Staiano, and Samuele Maria Marcora. "Talking Yourself Out of Exhaustion: The Effects of Self-Talk on Endurance Performance." *Medicine & Science in Sports & Exercise* 46, no. 5 (2014): 998–1007.

Borg, G. A. "Psychophysical Bases of Perceived Exertion." *Medicine & Science in Sports & Exercise* 14, no. 5 (1982): 377–381.

Boya, Manhal, Tom Foulsham, Florentina Hettinga, David Parry, Emily Williams, Hollie Jones, Andrew Sparks, David Marchant, Paul Ellison, Craig Bridge, Lars McNaughton, and Dominic Micklewright. "Information Acquisition Differences Between Experienced and Novice Time Trial Cyclists." *Medicine & Science in Sports & Exercise* 49, no. 9 (September 2017): 1884–1898.

Brehm, J. W., and E. A. Self. "Intensity of Motivation." *Annual Review of Psychology* 40 (1989): 109–131.

Brick, Noel, Mark J. Campbell, and Tadhg Macintyre. "Metacognitive Processes in the Self-Regulation of Performance in Elite Distance Runners." *Psychology of Sport and Exercise* 19 (February 2015): 1–9.

Chiang, Ted. *Exhalation: Stories*. New York: Vintage, 2019.

Cona, Giorgia, Annachiara Cavazzana, Antonio Paoli, Giuseppe Marcolin, Alessandro Grainer, and Patrizia Silvia Bisiacchi. "It's a Matter of Mind! Cognitive Functioning Predicts the Athletic Performance in Ultra-marathon Runners." *PLOS One* 10, no. 7 (July 2015): e0132943.

Corbett, J. "An Analysis of the Pacing Strategies Adopted by Elite Athletes During Track Cycling." *International Journal of Sports Physiology and Performance* 4, no. 2 (2009): 195–205. https://doi.org/10.1123/ijspp.4.2.195.

Crawley, Michael. *Out of Thin Air: Running Wisdom and Magic from Above the Clouds in Ethiopia*. London: Bloomsbury, 2020.

Crust, Lee, and Peter J. Clough. "Developing Mental Toughness: From Research to Practice." *Journal of Sport Psychology in Action* 2, no. 1 (2011): 21–32.

Demarie, S., J. R. Pycke, A. Pizzuti, and V. Billat. "Pacing Strategy of 800 m and 1500 m Freestyle Swimming Finals in the World Championships According to the Performance in Males and Females of Different Age Groups." *Applied Science* 13 (2023): 10515.

de Morree, H. M., C. Klein, and S. M. Marcora. "Cortical Substrates of the Effects of Caffeine and Time-on-Task on Perception of Effort." *Journal of Applied Physiology* 117, no. 12 (2014): 1514–1523. https://doi.org/10.1152/japplphysiol.00898.2013.

Diotaiuti, Pierluigi, Stefania Mancone, and Stefano Corrado. "Using Sports Tracker: Evidences on Dependence, Self-Regulatory Modes and Resilience in a Sample of Competitive Runners." *Psychology* 11, no. 1 (January 2020): 54–70.

do Carmo, Everton C., Renato Barroso, Andrew Renfree, Natalia R. da Silva, Saulo Gil, and Valmor Tricoli. "Affective Feelings and Perceived Exertion During a 10-km Time Trial and Head-to-Head Running Race." *International Journal of Sports Physiology and Performance* 11 (February 2020): 1–4.

Eaton, R. "Hunting Behaviour of the Cheetah." *Journal of Wildlife Management* 34 (1970): 56–67.

Edwards, Andrew, and Remco Polman. *Pacing in Sport and Exercise: A Psychophysiological Perspective*. New York: Nova, 2012.

Elbert, T., C. Pantev, C. Wienbruch, B. Rockstroh, and E. Taub. "Increased Cortical Representation of the Fingers of the Left Hand in String Players." *Science* 270, no. 5234 (October 1995): 305–307.

Elferink-Gemser, Marije T., and Florentina J. Hettinga. "Pacing and Self-Regulation: Important Skills for Talent Development in Endurance Sports." *International Journal of Sports Physiology and Performance* 12, no. 6 (July 2017): 831–835.

Eskreis-Winkler, Lauren, James J. Gross, and Angela L. Duckworth. "Grit: Sustained Self-Regulation in the Service of Superordinate Goals." In *Handbook of Self-Regulation: Research, Theory and Applications*, 3rd ed., edited by Kathleen D. Vohs and Roy F. Baumeister. New York: Guilford, 2016.

Farrell, P. A., J. H. Wilmore, E. F. Coyle, J. E. Billing, and D. L. Costill. "Plasma Lactate Accumulation and Distance Running Performance." *Medicine & Science in Sports & Exercise* 11, no. 4 (1979): 338–344.

García-González, Luis, M. Perla Moreno, Alberto Moreno, Alexander Gil, and Fernando del Villar. "Effectiveness of a Video-Feedback and Questioning Programme to Develop Cognitive Expertise in Sport." *PLOS One* 8, no. 12 (2013): e82270.

Garcin, Murielle, Jérémy B. J. Coquart, Sophie Robin, and Régis Matran. "Prediction of Time to Exhaustion in Competitive Cyclists from a Perceptually Based Scale." *Journal of Strength and Conditioning Research* 25, no. 5 (May 2011): 1393–1399.

Gendolla, Guido H. E., Mattie Tops, and Sandra L. Koole, eds. *Handbook of Biobehavioral Approaches to Self-Regulation*. New York: Springer, 2015.

Gilpatrick, Brendan. "Pacing Variability and Performance in a 100 Mile Ultra Marathon." Digital Commons, 2021. https://digitalcommons.library.umaine.edu/cgi/viewcontent.cgi?article=4545&context=etd.

Haney, T. A., Jr., and J. A. Mercer. "A Description of Variability of Pacing in Marathon Distance Running." *International Journal of Exercise Science* 4, no. 2 (2011): 133–140.

Hill, A. V., C. H. N. Long, and H. Lupton. "Muscular Exercise, Lactic Acid and the Supply and Utilisation of Oxygen: Parts I–III." *Proceedings of the Royal Society of London* 96, no. 679 (1924): 438–475. https://www.jstor.org/stable/81203.

Hirsh, Jacob B. "Decision-Making and Self-Regulation from a Social-Personality Neuroscience Perspective." Unpublished doctoral thesis, University of Toronto, 2010. https://tspace.library.utoronto.ca/bitstream/1807/32936/3/Hirsh_Jacob_B_20106_PhD_thesis.pdf.

Karahanoğlu, Armagan, Rúben Gouveia, Jasper Reenalda, and Geke Ludden. "How Are Sports-Trackers Used by Runners? Running-Related Data, Personal Goals, and Self-Tracking in Running." *Sensors* 21, no. 11 (2021): 3687.

Kirby, B. S., B. J. Winn, B. W. Wilkins, and A. M. Jones. "Interaction of Exercise Bioenergetics with Pacing Behavior Predicts Track Distance Running Performance." *Journal of Applied Physiology* 131, no. 5 (2021): 1532–1542. https://doi.org/10.1152/japplphysiol.00223.2021.

Kolsung, E. B., G. Ettema, and K. Skovereng. "Physiological Response to Cycling with Variable Versus Constant Power Output." *Frontiers in Physiology* 11 (2020): 1098. https://doi.org/10.3389/fphys.2020.01098.

Lambrick, Danielle, Alex Rowlands, Thomas Rowland, and Roger G. Eston. "Pacing Strategies of Inexperienced Children During Repeated 800 m Individual Time-Trials and Simulated Competition." *Pediatric Exercise Science* 25, no. 2 (May 2013): 198–211.

Latorre-Román, Pedro Ángel, Juan Francisco Fernández-Povedano, Jesús Salas-Sánchez, Felipe García-Pinillos, and Juan Antonio Párraga-Montilla. "The Ability of Runners to Identify Spatial and Temporal Variables of Speed During Endurance Running." *Motor Control* 24, no. 4 (July 2020): 499–511.

Lee, Tatia M. C., Chetwyn C. H. Chan, Ada W. S. Leung, Peter T. Fox, and Jia-Hong Gao. "Sex-Related Differences in Neural Activity During Risk Taking: An fMRI Study." *Cerebral Cortex* 19, no. 6 (June 2009): 1303–1312.

Le Meur, Y., T. Bernard, S. Dorel, C. R. Abbiss, G. Honnorat, J. Brisswalter, and C. Hausswirth. "Relationships Between Triathlon Performance and Pacing Strategy During the Run in an International Competition." *International Journal of Sports Physiology and Performance* 6, no. 2 (2011): 183–194. https://doi.org/10.1123/ijspp.6.2.183.

Liew, Guo Chen, Garry Kuan, Ngien Siong Chin, and Hairul Anuar Hashim. "Mental Toughness in Sport." *German Journal of Exercise and Sport Research* 49 (2019): 381–394.

Marcora, Samuele M. "Do We Really Need a Central Governor to Explain Brain Regulation of Exercise Performance?" *European Journal of Applied Physiology* 104, no. 5 (November 2008): 929–931.

Marcora, Samuele M., Walter Staiano, and V. Manning. "Mental Fatigue Impairs Physical Performance in Humans." *Journal of Applied Physiology* 106, no. 3 (2009): 857–864. https://doi.org/10.1152/japplphysiol.91324.2008.

Mauger, Alexis R., and Nick Sculthorpe. "A New VO$_2$max Protocol Allowing Self-Pacing in Maximal Incremental Exercise." *British Journal of Sports Medicine* 46, no. 1 (January 2012): 59–63. https://doi.org/10.1136/bjsports-2011-090006.

Méndez-Alonso, David, Jose Antonio Prieto-Saborit, Jose Ramón Bahamonde, and Estíbaliz Jiménez-Arberás. "Influence of Psychological Factors on the Success of the Ultra-trail Runner." *International Journal of Environmental Research and Public Health* 18, no. 5 (March 2021): 2704.

Molinari, C. A., P. Bresson, F. Palacin, and V. Billat. "Pace Controlled by a Steady-State Physiological Variable Is Associated with Better Performance in a 3000 m Run." *International Journal of Environmental Research and Public Health* 18, no. 15 (2021): 7886. https://doi.org/10.3390/ijerph18157886.

Morales-Alamo, David, José Losa-Reyna, Rafael Torres-Peralta, Marcos Martin-Rincon, Mario Perez-Valera, David Curtelin, Jesús Gustavo Ponce-González, Alfredo Santana, and José A. L. Calbet. "What Limits Performance during Whole-Body Incremental Exercise to Exhaustion in Humans?" *Journal of Physiology* 593, no. 20 (October 2015): 4631–4648.

Murakami, Haruki. *What I Talk About When I Talk About Running: A Memoir.* New York: Vintage, 2008.

Nikolaidis, Pantelis T., and Beat Knechtle. "Pacing in Age Group Marathoners in the 'New York City Marathon.'" *Research in Sports Medicine* 26, no. 1 (January–March 2018): 86–99.

Noakes, T. D. "1996 J. B. Wolffe Memorial Lecture: Challenging Beliefs: Ex Africa semper aliquid novi." *Medicine & Science in Sports & Exercise* 29, no. 5 (1997): 571–590.

———. "Time to Move beyond a Brainless Exercise Physiology: The Evidence for Complex Regulation of Human Exercise Performance." *Applied Physiology, Nutrition and Metabolism* 36, no. 1 (2011): 23–35. https://doi.org/10.1139/H10-082.

O'Leary, Thomas J., Johnny Collett, Ken Howells, and Martyn G. Morris. "High but Not Moderate-Intensity Endurance Training Increases Pain Tolerance: A Randomised Trial." *European Journal of Applied Physiology* 117, no. 11 (November 2017): 2201–2210.

Olympics.com. "Sport and Education Are a Winning Combination." Accessed February 6, 2024. https://olympics.com/athlete365/career/sport-and-education-are-a-winning-combination/.

Parshad, R. D., S. J. McGregor, M. A. Busa, J. D. Skufca, and E. Bollt. "A Statistical Approach to the Use of Control Entropy Identifies Differences in Constraints of Gait in Highly Trained versus Untrained Runners." *Mathematical Biosciences and Engineering* 9, no. 1 (2012): 123–145. https://doi.org/10.3934/mbe.2012.9.123.

Pettersen, S. D., P. M. Aslaksen, and S. A. Pettersen. "Pain Processing in Elite and High-Level Athletes Compared to Non-athletes." *Frontiers in Psychology* 11 (2020): 1908. https://doi.org/10.3389/fpsyg.2020.01908.

Scherr, Johannes, Bernd Wolfarth, Jeffrey W. Christle, Axel Pressler, Stefan Wagenpfeil, and Martin Halle. "Associations Between Borg's Rating of Perceived Exertion and Physiological Measures of Exercise Intensity." *European Journal of Applied Physiology* 113, no. 1 (January 2013): 147–155.

Scruton, Adrian, James Baker, Justin Roberts, Itay Basevitch, Viviane Merzbach, and Dan Gordon. "Pacing Accuracy During an Incremental Step Test in Adolescent Swimmers." *Open Access Journal of Sports Medicine* 6 (2015): 249–257.

Seabury, T., D. Benton, and H. A. Young. "Interoceptive Differences in Elite Sprint and Long-Distance Runners: A Multidimensional Investigation." *PLOS One* 18, no. 1 (2023): e0278067. https://doi.org/10.1371/journal.pone.0278067.

Skorski, S., O. Faude, K. Rausch, and T. Meyer. "Reproducibility of Pacing Profiles in Competitive Swimmers." *International Journal of Sports Medicine* 34, no. 2 (February 2013): 152–157.

Smyth, Barry. "Fast Starters and Slow Finishers: A Large-Scale Data Analysis of Pacing at the Beginning and End of the Marathon for Recreational Runners." *Journal of Sports Analytics* 4, no. 3 (2018): 229–242.

Smyth, Barry, and Aonghus Lawlor. "Longer Disciplined Tapers Improve Marathon Performance for Recreational Runners." *Frontiers in Sports and Active Living* 3 (2021): 735220.

Viana, Bruno Ferreira, Flávio Oliveira Pires, Allan Inoue, Dominic Micklewright, and Tony Meireles Santos. "Correlates of Mood and RPE During Multi-lap Off-Road Cycling." *Applied Psychophysiology and Biofeedback* 41, no. 1 (March 2016): 1–7.

Walsh, Vincent. "Is Sport the Brain's Biggest Challenge?" *Current Biology* 24, no. 18 (2014): R859–R860.

Weir, J. P., T. W. Beck, J. T. Cramer, and T. J. Housh. "Is Fatigue All in Your Head? A Critical Review of the Central Governor Model." *British Journal of Sports Medicine* 40, no. 7 (2006): 573–586.

Wiersma, Rikstje, Inge K. Stoter, Chris Visscher, Florentina J. Hettinga, and Marije T. Elferink-Gemser. "Development of 1500-m Pacing Behavior in Junior Speed Skaters: A Longitudinal Study." *International Journal of Sports Physiology and Performance* 12, no. 9 (October 2017): 1224–1231.

Wiggins, Bradley. *My Hour*. London: Vintage, 2015.

Wittekind, A. L., D. Micklewright, and R. Beneke. "Teleoanticipation in All-Out Short-Duration Cycling." *British Journal of Sports Medicine* 45, no. 2 (2011): 114–119. https://doi.org/10.1136/bjsm.2009.061580.

ABOUT THE AUTHOR

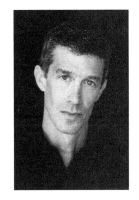

Matt Fitzgerald is an acclaimed endurance sports author, coach, and nutritionist. His many books include *Pain & Performance*, *The Comeback Quotient*, and *80/20 Running*. Matt has also written for a number of leading sports and fitness publications, including *Runner's World* and *Triathlete*, and for popular web sites such as outsideonline.com and nbcnews.com.

Matt is cofounder of 80/20 Endurance, the world's premier endurance sports training brand, where athletes can access training plans, videos, and other invaluable resources and inspiration, including a regular 80/20 Endurance podcast and blog. He also codirects the Coaches of Color Initiative, a nonprofit program that seeks to improve diversity in endurance coaching.

A lifelong endurance athlete, Matt speaks frequently at events throughout the United States and internationally and hosts Dream Run Camp, a prostyle residential training camp for runners of all abilities based in Flagstaff, Arizona.